A MANUAL OF
INTENSIVE CARE

A MANUAL OF
INTENSIVE CARE

Vinod Kumar Singh
MD MRCP FRCA FFICM
Assistant Professor
Department of Anesthesiology and Perioperative Medicine
University of Alabama at Birmingham (UAB) School of Medicine
Birmingham, Alabama, USA

Forewords
Keith A (Tony) Jones
Arun K Gupta

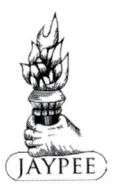

The Health Sciences Publisher
New Delhi | London | Panama

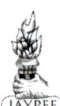 **Jaypee Brothers Medical Publishers (P) Ltd**

Headquarters

Jaypee Brothers Medical Publishers (P) Ltd
4838/24, Ansari Road, Daryaganj
New Delhi 110 002, India
Phone: +91-11-43574357
Fax: +91-11-43574314
Email: jaypee@jaypeebrothers.com

Overseas Offices

J.P. Medical Ltd
83 Victoria Street, London
SW1H 0HW (UK)
Phone: +44 20 3170 8910
Fax: +44 (0)20 3008 6180
Email: info@jpmedpub.com

Jaypee-Highlights Medical Publishers Inc
City of Knowledge, Bld. 235, 2nd Floor, Clayton
Panama City, Panama
Phone: +1 507-301-0496
Fax: +1 507-301-0499
Email: cservice@jphmedical.com

Jaypee Brothers Medical Publishers (P) Ltd
17/1-B Babar Road, Block-B, Shaymali
Mohammadpur, Dhaka-1207
Bangladesh
Mobile: +08801912003485
Email: jaypeedhaka@gmail.com

Jaypee Brothers Medical Publishers (P) Ltd
Bhotahity, Kathmandu
Nepal
Phone: +977-9741283608
Email: kathmandu@jaypeebrothers.com

Website: www.jaypeebrothers.com
Website: www.jaypeedigital.com

© 2017, Jaypee Brothers Medical Publishers

The views and opinions expressed in this book are solely those of the original contributor(s)/author(s) and do not necessarily represent those of editor(s) of the book.

All rights reserved. No part of this publication may be reproduced, stored or transmitted in any form or by any means, electronic, mechanical, photocopying, recording or otherwise, without the prior permission in writing of the publishers.

All brand names and product names used in this book are trade names, service marks, trademarks or registered trademarks of their respective owners. The publisher is not associated with any product or vendor mentioned in this book.

Medical knowledge and practice change constantly. This book is designed to provide accurate, authoritative information about the subject matter in question. However, readers are advised to check the most current information available on procedures included and check information from the manufacturer of each product to be administered, to verify the recommended dose, formula, method and duration of administration, adverse effects and contraindications. It is the responsibility of the practitioner to take all appropriate safety precautions. Neither the publisher nor the author(s)/editor(s) assume any liability for any injury and/or damage to persons or property arising from or related to use of material in this book.

This book is sold on the understanding that the publisher is not engaged in providing professional medical services. If such advice or services are required, the services of a competent medical professional should be sought.

Every effort has been made where necessary to contact holders of copyright to obtain permission to reproduce copyright material. If any have been inadvertently overlooked, the publisher will be pleased to make the necessary arrangements at the first opportunity.

Inquiries for bulk sales may be solicited at: jaypee@jaypeebrothers.com

A Manual of Intensive Care

First Edition: **2017**

ISBN: 978-93-5270-085-1

Printed at Rajkamal Electric Press, Plot No. 2, Phase-IV, Kundli, Haryana.

Dedicated to

My wife, Sipu who remains always my inspiration
My sons, Ishaan and Ryaan, the joys of my life
My parents and in-laws, who have always supported me

Foreword

Ever since the days of Florence Nightingale, intensive care has been evolving as a specialty. We have seen a rapid expansion in intensive care medicine over the last decade. It is a very complex field that combines the skills and knowledge from almost all the specialties in medicine. When a patient is unstable anywhere in the hospital, patients and physicians look for answers from the intensive care team. This makes the specialty highly satisfying. As the specialty spreads globally, new advances are seen on a daily basis. The manual, divided into 20 chapters, has been excellently planned to include all the topics relevant to the practice of intensive care medicine encompassing the recent advances. This book can be used as the bedside management of patients by the students and nurses alike. The chapters contains 'Golden tips' and 'Further readings' that makes it unique. The readers can explore the subject in more detail with this feature. I wish Dr Singh all the success with this book and sincerely hope that this book will be utilized widely in the field of intensive care medicine.

Keith A (Tony) Jones
MBBS MD
Professor and Alfred Habeeb Endowed Chair
Department of Anesthesiology
and Perioperative Medicine
University of Alabama School of Medicine
Birmingham, Alabama, USA

Foreword

The expansion of the specialty of intensive care medicine has captured the interest of the healthcare professionals worldwide. Our ability to combine clinical practice, based on a solid platform of basic science and technological advances, makes intensive care medicine an attractive and exciting specialty which has the potential to have a major impact on patient outcomes now and in the future.

The key to the delivery of high quality intensive care is in the education and training of healthcare staff at both the undergraduate and postgraduate levels. Dr Singh combines his passion for education with his expertise in intensive care in producing this manual. It will be an excellent companion to students and residents alike, providing the core knowledge which the practicing intensivist will need to deliver a safe and informed clinical care.

The chapters in the manual are well thought out to encompass all the areas of practice commonly seen in the ICU and make a quick and succinct reference which covers the key aspects of the subject matter. It is an ideal text to have 'on the shelf' in the ICU ward with some very useful features within chapters, such as the 'Golden tips' which highlight key aspects of a particular subject.

I hope readers of this manual find it interesting, informative and enjoyable. Most of all, I hope this manual will stimulate readers to follow a career in intensive care medicine—a fascinating, challenging and most rewarding specialty.

Arun K Gupta
MBBS MA PhD FFICM FRCA FHEA
Director of Postgraduate Education
Academic Health Sciences Centre
Cambridge University Health Partners
Director of the Addenbrooke's Simulation Centre
Consultant in Anaesthesia and Neurointensive Care
Cambridge University Hospitals
Associate Lecturer, University of Cambridge
Cambridge, UK

Preface

Intensive care medicine is rapidly gaining upfront position in modern medical care. Intensive care covers the knowledge, experience, expertise and much more from all the fields of medicine and surgery. Technically, intensive care specialty is on evidence-based medicine that demands knowledge of all and every medical skills at once. Doctors learning this art of medicine require quick reference to a wide variety of ailments encountered in critical care practice.

This book covers the essential topics related to intensive care medicine and emergency management of critically ill patients. Simplicity of language and elaborated illustrations and diagrams make this book easily readable. References are provided for further reading for the related topics. One of the highlights of this book is an easy explanation of procedures and techniques relevant to intensive care practice.

This book is presented in a way appropriate to the medical students and residents, physicians already working in the field of intensive care medicine and those who are interested in critical care medicine as a career. This book can also be used by the nursing staff for their curriculum and training as well as a quick reference while caring for the critically ill patients not only in the intensive care unit, but also the patients on general wards. This book will also help students taking their examinations in critical care medicine.

Regular use of this book will definitely add to the better outcomes for the critically ill patients. This book gives a very good overview of critical care medicine and intensive care in a systematic format, while providing easy readability for doctors and healthcare professionals at the same time.

Vinod Kumar Singh

Acknowledgments

I would like to thank:
- Dr Kazim Momin.
- My all friends and well-wishers, for their best wishes.
- Shri Jitendar P Vij (Group Chairman), Mr Ankit Vij (Group President) and their staff of M/s Jaypee Brothers Medical Publishers (P) Ltd, New Delhi, India, for publishing the book well in time.

Contents

1. **Monitoring and Procedures in Intensive Care**   1
   Arterial Line Insertion and Pressure Monitoring   1
   Central Line Insertion and Pressure Monitoring   2
   Pulse Oximetry   4
   End-tidal Carbon Dioxide Measurement   5
   Intracranial Pressure Monitoring   7
   Pulmonary Artery Catheter Placement   9
   Intercostal Drain Insertion   12

2. **Basic Care in ICU**   15
   Anxiety and Sedation   15
   Depression   18
   Delirium   19
   Pain   20
   Nutrition in Intensive Care Unit   21
   Blood Sugar Control in ICU   23
   Prevention of Gastric Ulcer in ICU   24
   Causes and Risks   24
   Thromboprophylaxis in ICU   26

3. **Cardiovascular System**   29
   Stable Angina Pectoris   29
   Unstable Angina   30
   Myocardial Infarction (ST Segment Elevation)   30
   Bradycardia and Heart Block   32
   Atrial Fibrillation   33
   Supraventricular Tachycardia   35
   Management   36
   Ventricular Tachycardia   37
   Mitral Valve   38
   Aortic Valve   39
   Cardiac Tamponade   40
   Congestive Cardiac Failure   42
   Aortic Dissection   43
   Hypertensive Crisis   44

4. **Renal Disorders in Intensive Care**   46
   Acute Kidney Injury   46
   Renal Failure in Intensive Care Unit   48
   Acute Tubular Necrosis   49
   Rhabdomyolysis   50
   Hepatorenal Syndrome   52
   Pulmonary Renal Syndromes   53
   Renal Replacement in Intensive Care Unit   54

5. Essential Neurology — 58

Guillain-Barre Syndrome 58
Myasthenia Gravis 60
Muscular Dystrophy 61
Critical Illness Polyneuropathy 63
Critical Illness Myopathy 64
Head Injury 64
Intracranial Hypertension 67
Stroke 69
Subarachnoid Hemorrhage 71
Altered Sensorium 73
Coma 75
Status Epilepticus 77

6. Fluid and Electrolyte Disorders — 79

Hypernatremia 79
Hyponatremia 80
Hyperkalemia 81
Hypokalemia 82
Hypercalcemia 83
Hypocalcemia 84
Hypermagnesemia 85
Hypomagnesemia 86
Hyperphosphatemia 86
Hypophosphatemia 87
Hypervolemia 88
Hypovolemia 88

7. Acid and Base Disorders — 90

Metabolic Acidosis 90
Metabolic Alkalosis 91
Respiratory Acidosis 92
Respiratory Alkalosis 93
Mixed Acid-Base Disturbances 94

8. Shock — 96

Sepsis and Septic Shock 96
Cardiogenic Shock 97
Hypovolemic Shock 98
Obstructive Shock 99
Neurogenic Shock 100
Anaphylactic Shock 101

9. Endocrine Problems in ICU — 103

Diabetic Ketoacidosis 103
Hyperosmolar Non-ketotic Diabetic Coma 104
Hypoglycemia 105
Adrenal Failure 105
Cushing's Syndrome 106
Thyrotoxicosis 107
Myxedema due to Hypothyroidism 108

10. Oncological Emergencies — 110
Acute Leukemia 110
Tumor Lysis Syndrome 111
Superior Vena Cava Syndrome 111

11. Pregnancy and ICU — 113
Preeclampsia and Eclampsia 113
Acute Fatty Liver of Pregnancy 114
Amniotic Fluid Embolism 114
Septic Abortion 115
Pregnancy and Asthma 115
Pulmonary Edema in Pregnancy 116

12. Gastrointestinal Diseases — 118
Small Bowel Obstruction 118
Large Bowel Obstruction 119
Paralytic Ileus 120
Upper Gastrointestinal Bleeding 121
Lower Gastrointestinal Bleeding 122
Gastritis 122
Peptic Ulcer Disease 123
Variceal Bleeding 124
Pancreatitis 124
Acute Hepatic Failure 125
Ascites 126
Diarrhea 127
Acute Cholangitis 128

13. Poisonings — 130
Organophosphorus Poisoning 130
Paracetamol Overdose 130
Salicylate Overdose 132
Tricyclic Antidepressant Overdose 132
Beta-blocker Overdose 133
Calcium-channel Blocker Overdose 133
Digitalis Toxicity 134
Methanol Poisoning 134
Alcohol Withdrawal 135
Benzodiazepine Withdrawal 136
Opioid Withdrawal 136
Opioid Overdose 137
Carbon Monoxide Poisoning 138
Snakebite 139

14. Environmental Injuries — 141
Heatstroke 141
Hypothermia 141
Frostbite 142
Near-drowning 143
Electrical Injuries 144
Acute Inhalational Injury 144

15. Skin Diseases in ICU — 146
- Measles 146
- Chicken Pox 147
- Toxic Shock Syndrome 148
- Drug Reactions 148
- Steven Johnson Syndrome 149
- Toxic Epidermal Necrolysis Syndrome 149
- Disseminated Intravascular Coagulation 150
- Pemphigus Vulgaris 151
- Graft versus Host Disease 152
- *Candida* Infection 152
- Meningococcal Infection 153

16. Rheumatology — 155
- Systemic Lupus Erythematosus 155
- Scleroderma/Systemic Sclerosis 156
- Vasculitis 157
- Antiphospholipid Syndrome 158

17. Infections — 159
- Pyrexia of Unknown Origin in ICU 159
- Infection in Immunocompromized Patients 160
- Sepsis 160
- Neutropenic Sepsis 161
- Infective Endocarditis 161
- Urinary Tract Infections 162
- Community-acquired Pneumonia 163
- Hospital-acquired Pneumonia 163
- Intravenous Catheter Related Bloodstream Infections 164
- Intra-abdominal Infections 165
- *Clostridium difficile*-associated Diarrhea 165
- Bacterial Meningitis 166
- Encephalitis 167
- *Mycobacterium tuberculosis* 167
- *Pneumocystis jirovecii* Pneumonia 168
- Tetanus 168
- Botulism 169
- Necrotizing Fasciitis 169
- Toxic Shock Syndrome 170
- Systemic Candidiasis 170

18. Hematological Disorders — 172
- Bleeding in ICU 172
- Thrombocytopenia 173
- Qualitative Platelet Dysfunction 174
- Heparin-induced Thrombocytopenia 174
- Acquired Coagulopathies 175
- Inherited Coagulopathy 175
- Warfarin Toxicity 176
- Red Cell Transfusion 176
- Plasma Transfusions 177
- Transfusion Reactions 178

19. Special Considerations in ICU — 179
- Brain Death 179
- Burns and Its Management 179
- Patients with Chronic Renal Failure 181
- Pregnant Patients in ICU 181
- Transplant Patients in ICU 182
- Care of Elderly Patients 182
- Obese Patients 183

20. Respiratory Disorders and Management in ICU — 185
- Pneumothorax 185
- Pleural Effusion 186
- Positive End-expiratory Pressure 187
- Noninvasive Ventilation 188
- Invasive Ventilation 189
- Acute Severe Asthma 189
- Ventilation in Acute Severe Asthma 190
- Chronic Obstructive Pulmonary Disease 190
- Pulmonary Thromboembolism 191
- Air Embolism 192
- Obstructive Sleep Apnea 193
- Obesity Hypoventilation Syndrome 193
- Aspiration Pneumonia 194
- Ventilator-associated Pneumonia 194
- Hypoxia 195
- Hypercapnia 196
- Hemoptysis 196
- Acute Respiratory Distress Syndrome 197
- Ventilation in ARDS 197

Index 199

PLATE 1

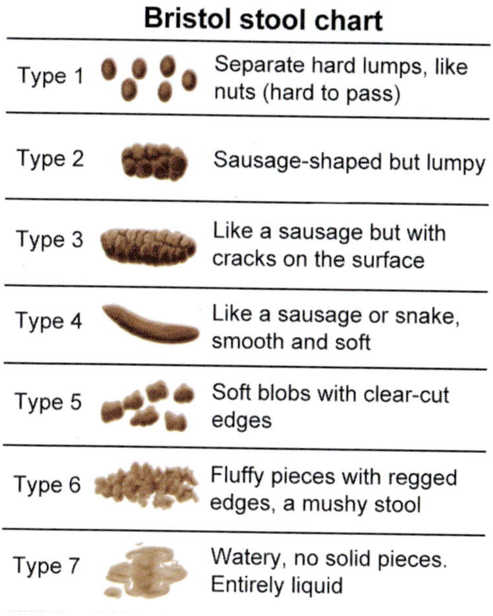

Bristol stool chart

Type 1		Separate hard lumps, like nuts (hard to pass)
Type 2		Sausage-shaped but lumpy
Type 3		Like a sausage but with cracks on the surface
Type 4		Like a sausage or snake, smooth and soft
Type 5		Soft blobs with clear-cut edges
Type 6		Fluffy pieces with regged edges, a mushy stool
Type 7		Watery, no solid pieces. Entirely liquid

FIGURE 12.4: Bristol stool chart is used for defining the type of stools

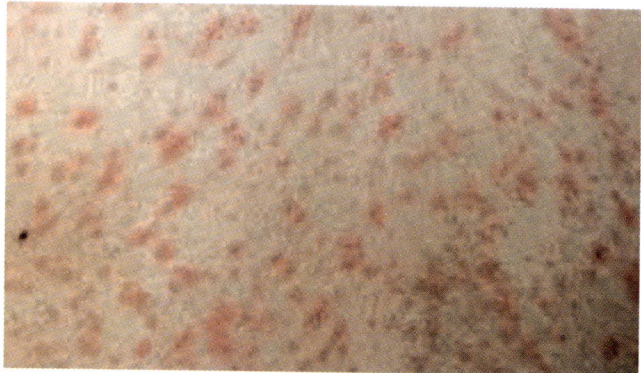

FIGURE 15.1: Measles rash

PLATE 2

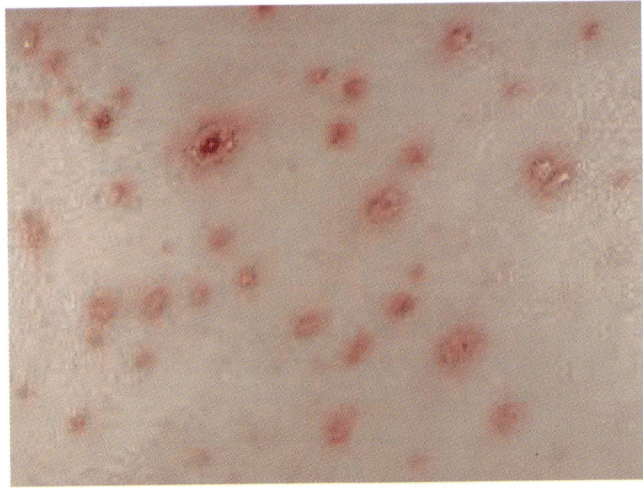

FIGURE 15.2: Chicken pox rash

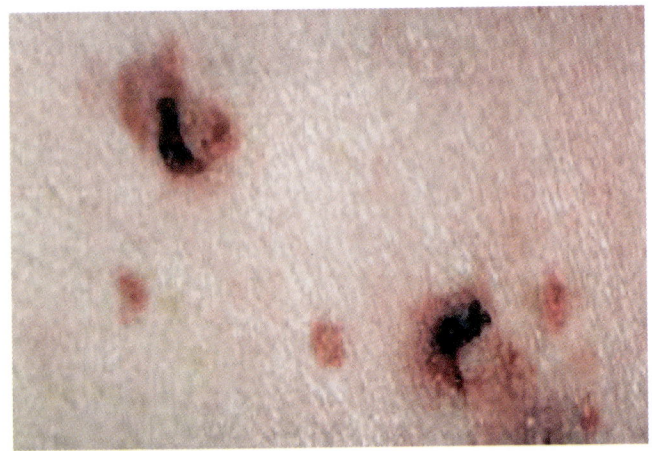

FIGURE 15.3: Pemphigus vulgaris

PLATE 3

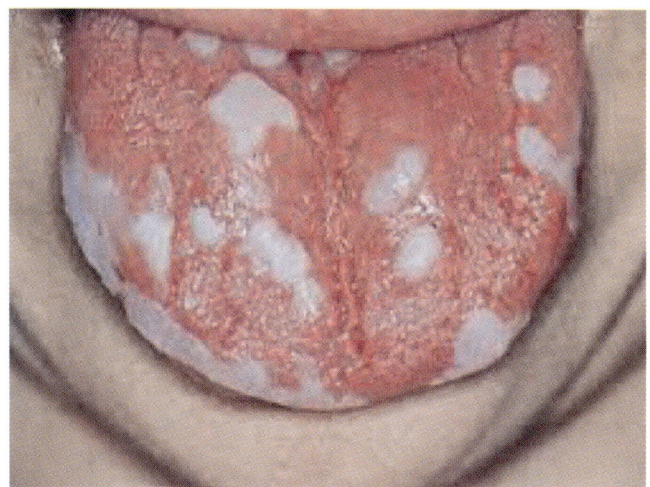

FIGURE 15.4: Oral condidiasis

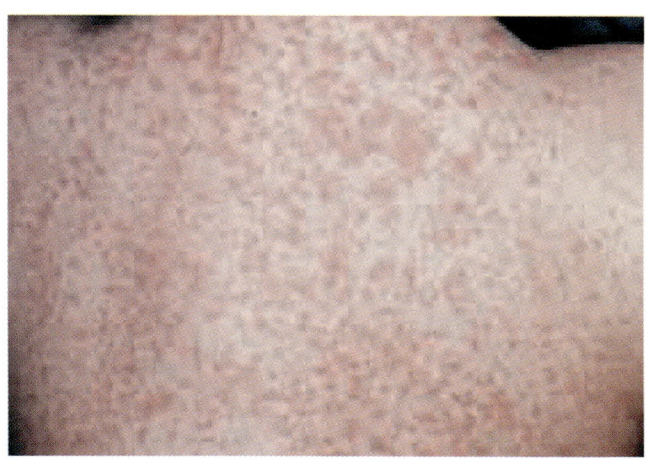

FIGURE 15.5: Meningococcal rash

CHAPTER 1

Monitoring and Procedures in Intensive Care

Arterial Line Insertion and Pressure Monitoring

Arterial catheters are used commonly in critical care patients to obtain blood, measure the blood pressure directly and estimate the cardiac output. As this is an invasive procedure, caution should be exercised and complications should be avoided.

Indications

- Blood pressure monitoring in hypotension, hypertensive episodes, major surgeries and guiding vasoactive medication therapy
- Frequent blood gas or laboratory measurements in sick patients
- Monitoring cardiac output by softwares like LiDCO (lithium dilution cardiac output).

Insertion

Identify the palpable artery. Radial artery is the most commonly used. The collateral flow can be checked by occluding the ulnar artery. The arm is immobilized and area is aseptically cleaned and prepared. Local anesthetic can be used to numb the area. Ultrasound can also be used for locating the artery. Various techniques are used depending on the user experience and include separate-guidewire, integral guidewire, direct puncture or the seldinger technique.

Contraindications and Complications

Coagulopathy and use of thrombolytic agents are relative contraindications.
Complications include:
- Hematoma and bleeding
- Pain and bruising
- Thrombosis and embolism
- Infection
- Air embolism and blood loss.

Pressure Monitoring

Arterial pressure monitoring remains the gold standard of blood pressure measurement (Fig. 1.1). It correlates well with indirect measurements in healthy patients, but not so much in sick patients or patients with calcified arteries, arrhythmias or certain medications. The arterial trace accuracy depends on a number of factors though including proper calibration, position of the transducer and also the damping coefficient and resonant frequency of the system.

Golden Tips

- Use of ultrasound can increase the success rate and reduce time taken for catheterization
- Local anesthetic usage reduces pain without reducing the chance of success
- Arterial catheters should not be replaced routinely unless there are signs of infection or catheter failure.

Central Line Insertion and Pressure Monitoring

Central venous catheter placement is common in the ICU settings. It is an invasive procedure with higher rate of infections and more serious complications compared to the arterial line.

Indications

- Administration of medications such as vasoactive medications, parenteral nutrition, chemotherapy, concentrated electrolytes like potassium
- Renal replacement therapy (hemodialysis/hemofiltration) and plasmapheresis
- Hemodynamic monitoring in the form of central venous pressure, central venous oxygen saturations and insertion of pulmonary artery catheter
- Transvenous pacing and stent placement
- Poor venous access.

Contraindications

- Coagulopathy
- Local infection

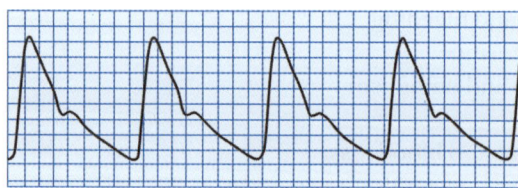

FIGURE 1.1: Arterial line trace

- ❏ Bleeding diasthesis
- ❏ Already indwelling catheter presence are all relative contraindications.

Method

The common sites of insertion are internal jugular, subclavian and femoral veins. The catheter can be placed percutaneously or surgically. They can also be tunnelled or non-tunnelled. They come in various sizes and number of lumens. Another type is the peripherally inserted central catheter (PiCC) that is generally inserted in the basilic/cephalic vein and ends in the right atrium/superior vena cava. This device has lower complication rate and better patient satisfaction. The device to be inserted should be selected carefully based on the need of the particular patient and the need reviewed daily.

The common sites for cannulation include jugular vein, subclavian vein and femoral vein. There is little difference in the mechanical or infective complications with jugular or subclavian vein with subclavian access having higher mechanical complications while jugular vein access having higher infective complications. If a patient has respiratory compromise, jugular route is preferred and subclavian site is generally avoided in coagulopathy. Femoral site may have higher infection risk compared to jugular or subclavian route, more so with increased BMI. After consent, monitoring and sterile prepping of the site, the patient should be positioned such that the vein is prominent (head down for jugular vein if tolerated by patient). Ultrasound may be used here if available in a sterile fashion. Seldinger technique is generally used for cannulation. Local anesthetic is used to numb the skin and extra sedation/analgesics given as appropriate. Vein is then cannulated to get the blood back following which the guidewire is inserted. Needle is then removed, skin nicked with a blade and dilated using the dilator. The catheter is then inserted over the guidewire and guidewire removed. The catheter is then secured to the skin after all the ports have been aspirated and flushed. A sterile transparent dressing is applied and the position checked with a chest X-ray in cases of subclavian and jugular routes.

Complications

- ❏ Hematoma and bleeding
- ❏ Arterial puncture
- ❏ Arrythmias due to guidewire stimulating the heart
- ❏ Pneumothorax/hemothorax
- ❏ Injury to nerves, thoracic duct, other structures around the area
- ❏ Loss of guidewire into the vein.

Golden Tips

- ❏ Use of ultrasound reduces the complication rates and is recommended whenever available

- Jugular and subclavian routes can be used unless specific contraindications exist. Femoral route may have higher infection rates
- The need for central venous access should be reviewed daily.

Pulse Oximetry

Pulse oximetry has become a vital part of monitoring in the recent years. This is a non-invasive method of estimating the arterial hemoglobin concentration while avoiding the requirements of arterial puncture and blood gas machine for calculation of dissolved oxygen in the blood.

Concepts

Photoplethysmography is used to calculate the oxygenation of hemoglobin using the Beer–Lambert law. Two different wavelengths are used to differentiate between deoxyhemoglobin and oxyhemoglobin. Deoxyhemoglobin absorbs light in the red band (600–750 nm), while oxyhemoglobin in the infrared (850–1000 nm). The relative absorbance is used to calculate the oxyhemoglobin saturation in percentage. The diodes in the probe emit at 660 and 940 nm and the probe is placed on the fingers or earlobes. This data is collected during pulsatile and non-pulsatile flow and then the noise is eliminated based on this. The pulse oximeter can also display the heart rate based on the pulsatile flow. The values are accurate from 70–100% range.

Uses

Any situation where there is a risk of variation in the saturations or chances of deterioration over time. This may include:
- Intensive care units, where the saturations can be followed instead of repeated arterial blood gas measurements
- Emergency departments for use in sick patients
- Intra- and peri-operatively to monitor the oxygenation of patients
- Sleep and exercise laboratories, conscious sedations, labor suites.

It has the benefit of providing the hemoglobin saturation rather than the dissolved oxygen content. As 98% of the oxygen is attached to hemoglobin, it offers a better indicator of oxygenation.

Limitations

- Poor perfusion may result in artifacts
- Motion artifacts, ambient light and electromagnetic radiations can all interfere with the readings
- Oxyhemoglobin, methemoglobin and carboxyhemoglobin can all be measured as oxyhemoglobin. Sickle hemoglobin can also cause variations in the reading to a lesser extent

- Skin pigmentation, nail polish and some dyes like methylene blue can also cause low oximetry readings
- Does not measure the CO_2 and hence ventilation status of the patient.
- There is a delay of several seconds which may be significant in neonates/pediatric patients
- Large decrease in dissolved oxygen will still not be detected with pulse oximetry as the dissociation curve only changes around 70 mm Hg.

Golden Tips

- Pulse oximetry gives the hemoglobin saturations compared to dissolved oxygen content from arterial gases
- It is a cheap, continuous and non-invasive method of monitoring patients status.

End-tidal Carbon Dioxide Measurement

Carbon dioxide monitoring or capnography/capnometry is a noninvasive way of monitoring the partial pressure of CO_2 in expired gases. This can be represented in the form of a number, change in color or a waveform (Fig. 1.2). Capnography can be used for a variety of clinical indications as discussed below and have become a standard part of monitoring in anesthesia and critical care.

Concepts

End tidal carbon dioxide measurement can be done by sidestream or mainstream systems. The measurement is done with qualitative methods or quantitative methods. Quantitative methods give the waveform (capnography) or a number (capnometry); while qualitative methods report a range by change in color by use of treated litmus paper. These are useful when confirmation of endotracheal tube placement is warranted. Capnography uses infrared waves for the measurements. This is absorbed by CO_2 in the breath and is displayed in the form of a wave or number.

The capnograph has various phases depending on the cycle of respiration. The first phase (with CO_2 close to 0) is the expiration where the dead space is being cleared. The ascending phase is when the alveolar gases start reaching the capnograph monitor. The next phase is the plateau phase of alveolar

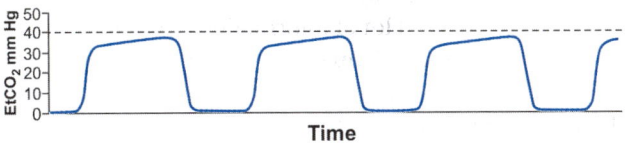

FIGURE 1.2: Normal capnogram

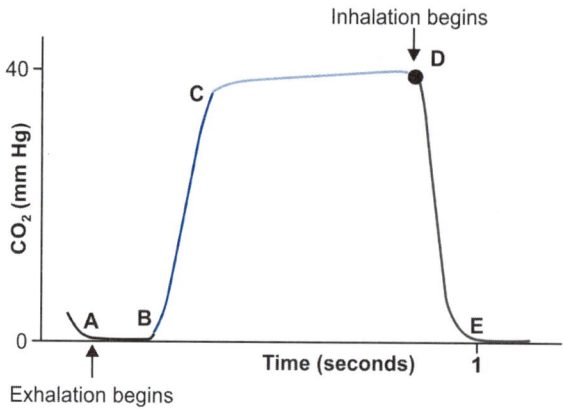

FIGURE 1.3: Phases of a normal capnogram

expiration which peaks towards the end (end-tidal CO_2) of the tidal breath. The number may be represented on the monitor and the final phase is the inspiratory phase where fresh air is breathed in. The end-tidal CO_2 may be very close to the arterial CO_2 ($PaCO_2$) in healthy patients, but can be below the $PaCO_2$ in diseased states like COPD, pulmonary embolism, pneumonia, etc.

Uses

- Correlation with $PaCO_2$ in health patients
- Verifying placement of endotracheal tube
- Titration and determination of ventilation adequacy
- Useful in transport of patients
- Diagnosing cardiac output drop (if the end-tidal CO_2 reduces suddenly)
- Calculation of respiratory rate and monitoring of sedated patients.

Limitations

- Cannot help in diagnosing the cause of ventilation problem
- There may be delay in getting the measurements in side-stream analysers while the mainstream analyzers may be bulky
- They should not be relied completely to represent $PaCO_2$ unless the patient is healthy with normal lung function.

Golden Tips

- End-tidal CO_2 monitoring may be qualitative or quantitative
- The capnograph can give a lot of information about the patient including presence of airway disease, adequacy of ventilation, respiratory rate, limited information on perfusion and metabolism and response to treatment
- It should be used in all patients with airway device in situ
- In patients undergoing sedation for a procedure, the side-stream monitor can be used for monitoring the respiratory rate.

Intracranial Pressure Monitoring

Neurological insult in the form of trauma, stroke, tumors and metabolic derangements can lead to increase in the intracranial pressure. Recognition and early treatment with the use of intracranial monitoring devices can be important in treating and reversing these conditions.

Concepts

The normal intracranial pressure is <15 mm Hg. As the intracranial compartment has a fixed volume, any change in any of its contents—blood, brain matter and cerebrospinal fluid will cause a rise in the intracranial pressure and affect organ perfusion and blood supply (Monro-Kellie doctrine). The cerebral perfusion pressure is important and is calculated from the intracranial pressure measurement.

CPP = MAP − ICP (Cerebral perfusion pressure = Mean arterial pressure − Intracranial pressure).

Cerebral perfusion pressure of more than 70 mm Hg is considered adequate and hence the mean arterial pressure is manipulated to keep the CPP at a reasonable level. ICP monitoring is hence useful in this calculation. Intracranial pressure can be measured by various devices and should be kept if possible below 20 mm Hg.

Devices

The use of ICP monitoring is to help the clinicians make adjustments to maintain the CPP. This can improve the patient outcome especially in trauma patients. CT scans are the preliminary diagnostic tools for such neurological insult and can demonstrate mass lesions, midline shifts and herniation of brain matter or hydrocephalus. This can point towards increased ICP, but cannot measure the actual value. Also ICP can be raised with normal CT scans too. Thus other types of devices are used for more direct measurement of ICP. These can be intraventricular, intraparenchymal, subarachnoid and epidural devices.

Intraventricular

Intraventricular monitors measure the pressure directly from the ventricles and are most reliable. They also have the benefit of draining the CSF to relieve the pressure, hence they have therapeutic role. Infections can occur and there is small chance of hemorrhage. They cannot be placed if the ventricles are small.

Intraparenchymal

Intraparenchymal monitors have a small transducer at their tip and are directly left in the brain parenchyma through a small drill (bolt). They are easy to place, have lower risk of infection and bleeding, but cannot be used to drain the CSF. They are useful when the ventricles are small.

Subarachnoid

Subarachnoid monitors are placed through the skull into the dura and the dura then perforated for communication with the transducer. They have low infection or hemorrhage rates, but can be unreliable and inaccurate.

Epidural

Epidural monitors are placed on the dura without piercing the dura. They can be unreliable too, but are more useful in patients with bleeding diasthesis.

Waves generated from the monitors can give an idea of the advanced pathology (Figs 1.4A to C). Pathological A waves are marked elevations in the ICP to 100 mm Hg lasting minutes to hours, B waves can be transient due to vasospasm and C waves are smaller changes related to respiration and cardiac activity.

Non-invasive methods for ICP estimation are also used in the form of transorbital sonography, transcranial Doppler, tympanic membrane displacement, intraocular pressure monitoring, tissue resonance analysis, etc.

Golden Tips

- ICP monitors are invasive monitors with increased chances of infection, hence should be placed in appropriately indicated situations
- Intraventricular drains have benefit of draining CSF to reduce pressure.

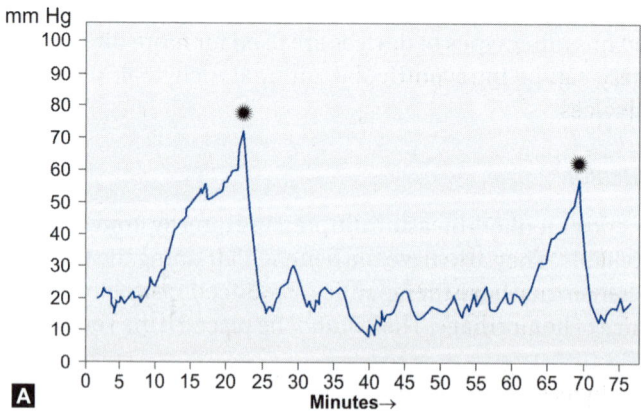

FIGURE 1.4A

Monitoring and Procedures in Intensive Care

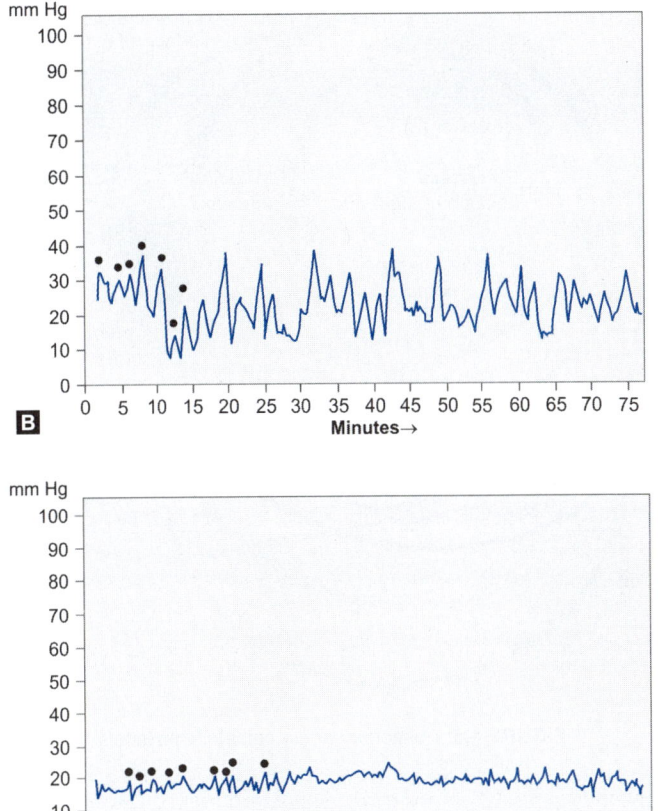

FIGURES 1.4B AND C

FIGURES 1.4A TO C: Intracranial pressure waves: (A) A waves (Plateau waves); (B) B waves; (C) C waves

Pulmonary Artery Catheter Placement

Flow directed pulmonary artery catheter has been the gold standard for cardiac output monitoring and estimation of right sided pressures for years. This technique has now slowly waned to give way to new non-invasive or semi-invasive methods of cardiac output monitoring like LiDCO and PiCCO.

Concepts

Hemodynamic data obtained from the correct placement of the pulmonary artery catheter (Fig. 1.5). This can give direct measurements of pressures from the right atrium, right ventricle, pulmonary artery and the pulmonary artery

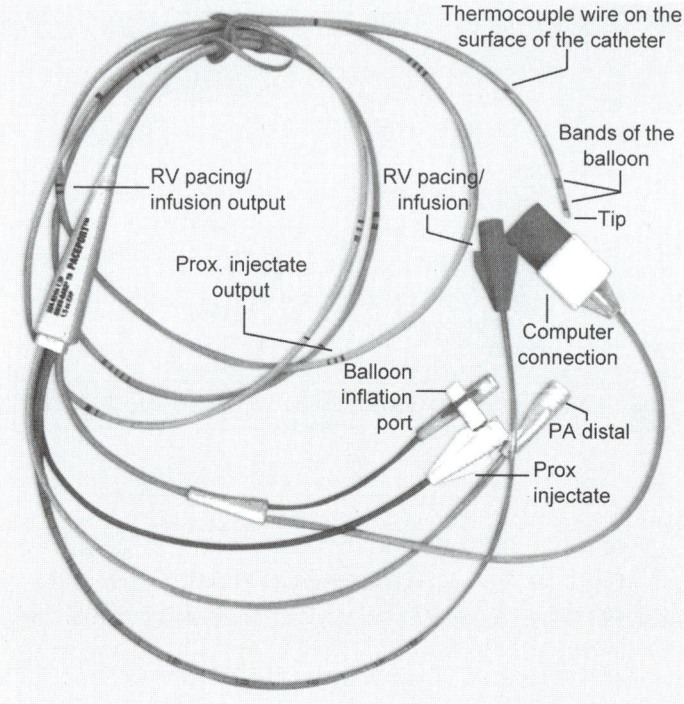

FIGURE 1.5: Pulmonary artery catheter with labels

wedge. Thermodilution technique may be used to estimate the cardiac output quite accurately and based on these measurements; data can be derived for pulmonary vascular and peripheral vascular resistance to guide vasoactive therapy. Blood gases obtained can give the mixed venous oxygen saturations for guiding fluid therapy too. This advantage of the catheters has not been shown to improve morbidity or mortality in various studies and the risks involved because of the invasive nature has made them less favorable compared to other techniques in many situations.

Placement of Catheter

The PA catheter is inserted in an aseptic technique through the introducer; which is a central venous line usually placed in the jugular or subclavian veins. The catheter is connected to the transducer to check the trace during insertion. Once the catheter is in the right atrium, the balloon at the tip of the catheter is inflated and the flow of blood should direct the catheter towards the pulmonary artery via the right ventricle. The waveform should continuously guide the operator about the position of the catheter (Fig. 1.6). Once the catheter is in the pulmonary artery branch, the balloon wedges and stops flow through the arteriole, hence equilibrating the pressure with the left atrium. This gives the

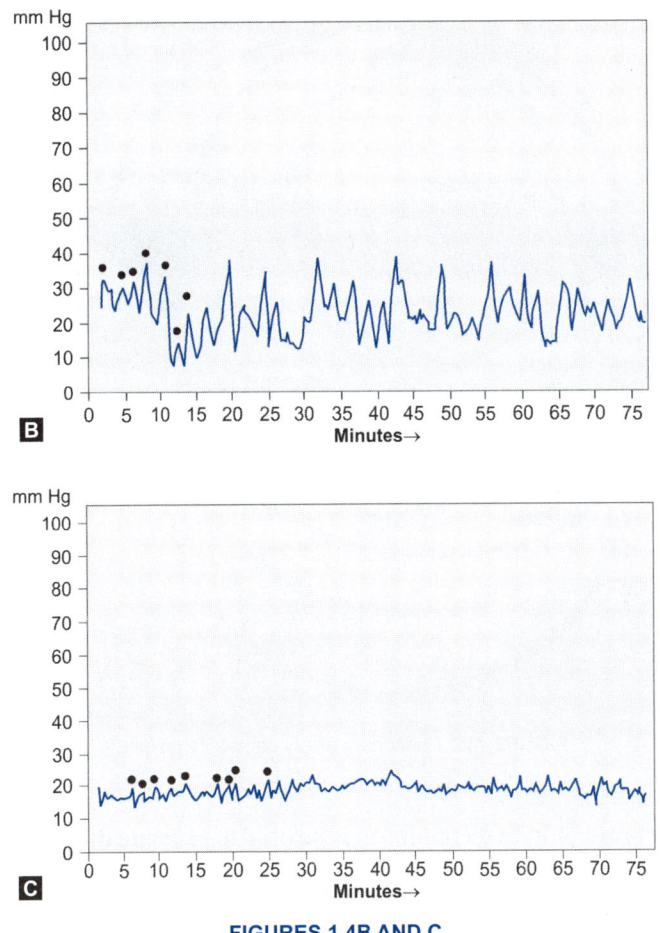

FIGURES 1.4B AND C

FIGURES 1.4A TO C: Intracranial pressure waves: (A) A waves (Plateau waves); (B) B waves; (C) C waves

Pulmonary Artery Catheter Placement

Flow directed pulmonary artery catheter has been the gold standard for cardiac output monitoring and estimation of right sided pressures for years. This technique has now slowly waned to give way to new non-invasive or semi-invasive methods of cardiac output monitoring like LiDCO and PiCCO.

Concepts

Hemodynamic data obtained from the correct placement of the pulmonary artery catheter (Fig. 1.5). This can give direct measurements of pressures from the right atrium, right ventricle, pulmonary artery and the pulmonary artery

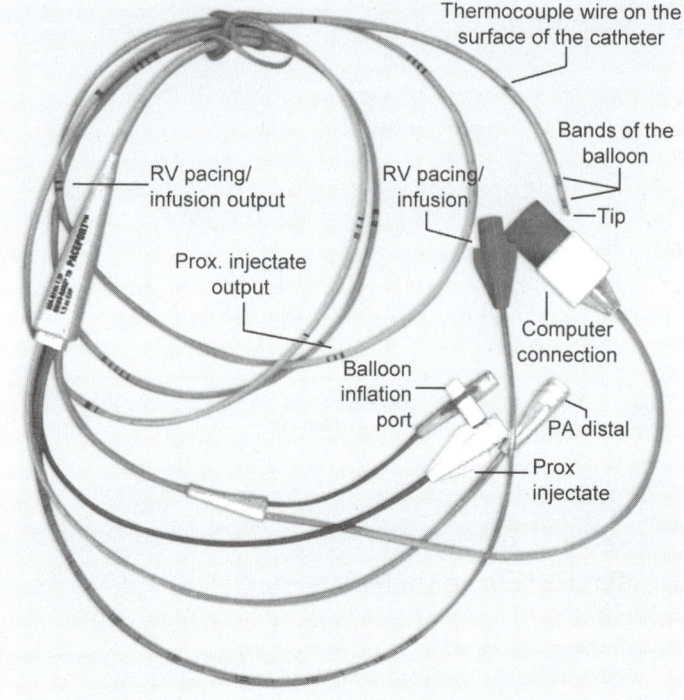

FIGURE 1.5: Pulmonary artery catheter with labels

wedge. Thermodilution technique may be used to estimate the cardiac output quite accurately and based on these measurements; data can be derived for pulmonary vascular and peripheral vascular resistance to guide vasoactive therapy. Blood gases obtained can give the mixed venous oxygen saturations for guiding fluid therapy too. This advantage of the catheters has not been shown to improve morbidity or mortality in various studies and the risks involved because of the invasive nature has made them less favorable compared to other techniques in many situations.

Placement of Catheter

The PA catheter is inserted in an aseptic technique through the introducer; which is a central venous line usually placed in the jugular or subclavian veins. The catheter is connected to the transducer to check the trace during insertion. Once the catheter is in the right atrium, the balloon at the tip of the catheter is inflated and the flow of blood should direct the catheter towards the pulmonary artery via the right ventricle. The waveform should continuously guide the operator about the position of the catheter (Fig. 1.6). Once the catheter is in the pulmonary artery branch, the balloon wedges and stops flow through the arteriole, hence equilibrating the pressure with the left atrium. This gives the

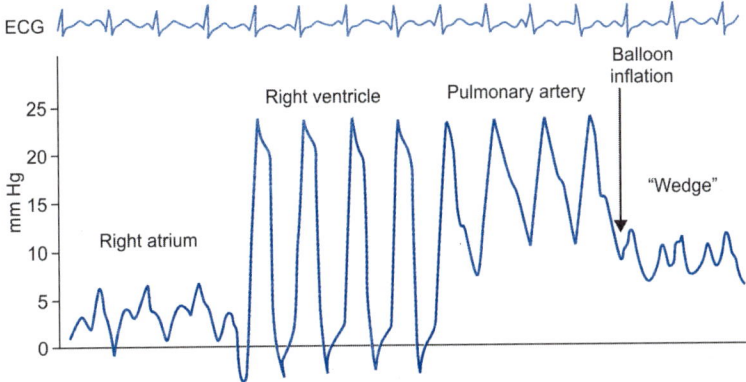

FIGURE 1.6: Waveform recorded with PA catheter as it trespasses various structures of the heart

estimation of the left heart pressures. Caution should be exercised in insertion and withdrawal of these catheters as serious complications can result including pulmonary artery rupture.

Complications and Precautions

All the complications associated with central line placement can occur while placing the introducer.

During floatation of the PA catheter:
- Atrial and ventricular tachycardia needing urgent intervention
- Vascular injury including pulmonary artery rupture
- Knotting of the catheter
- Misplacement
- Infection
- Valvular rupture/avulsion
- Pulmonary infarction
- Thrombus and embolism (including air embolism)
- Data interpretation and calibration issues.

Golden Tips

- Pulmonary artery catheters are slowly falling out of favor due to poor evidence of benefit and increased risk to the patients
- PA catheters provide direct measurement of a wide variety of hemodynamic parameters and may be useful if used appropriately
- Always deflate the balloon while withdrawing the catheter and inflate while advancing the catheter.

Intercostal Drain Insertion

Intercostal drain or tube thoracostomy is performed to drain air or fluid from the pleural space and rarely to introduce medications for chemotherapy or pleurodesis.

Indications and Contraindications

Indications

- Pneumothorax (spontaneous, iatrogenic, traumatic, tension or bronchopleural fistula)
- Hemothorax (trauma, postoperative, malignant)
- Pleural effusion (infection, empyema, malignant, chyle, parapneumonic effusions)
- Others: Pleurodesis, instillation of chemotherapeutic agents.

Contraindications/Cautions

- Coagulation abnormalities
- Anticoagulation
- Transudative effusions like cardiac failure, hepatic or renal failure.

Intracostal Drain Placement

Appropriate patient selection is important. If there is previous history of difficult placement, repeated infections (leading to fibrosis) or history of malignancy, caution should be exercised and ultrasound or CT-guidance obtained. Care must be taken with very large effusions where sudden removal of fluid can cause pulmonary edema. Appropriate size tube should be selected. Small tubes for simple pneumothorax and transudative effusions may be appropriate, but larger tubes are needed for empyema, blood, infected and exudative effusions. Similarly bronchopleural fistulas may need bigger tubes. Seldinger technique can be used depending on the indication and user experience.

Procedure should be explained to the patient, area prepared aseptically and local anesthetic used to reduce discomfort. The 4/5th intercostal space in the anterior/mid axillary line is preferred due to safety (safe triangle) (Fig. 1.7). Ultrasound can be helpful in deciding the site of insertion and depth. Patients arms can be placed above the head for better access. Skin incision is made parallel to intercostal space and subcutaneous tissue and muscles are dissected bluntly with forceps. The insertion should preferably be just above the rib to avoid the neurovascular bundle. Once close to the pleura, the forceps or clamp is used to go through the pleura after checking with a finger. The finger is sweeped to clear the space and check the lung for adhesions and other structures. The tube is then held with clamp/forceps and introduced through the tract and directed appropriately. For pneumothorax, the tube is directed anteriorly, while for hemothorax posteriorly. All the drainage holes should be

Monitoring and Procedures in Intensive Care 13

within the pleural space to avoid leaks and subcutaneous emphysema. Once the tube is in place, this should be connected to the closed seal system and sutured securely to the skin. Many different types of seals are available (Fig. 1.8). For better drainage, suction can be applied too (0 to -40 cm H_2O).

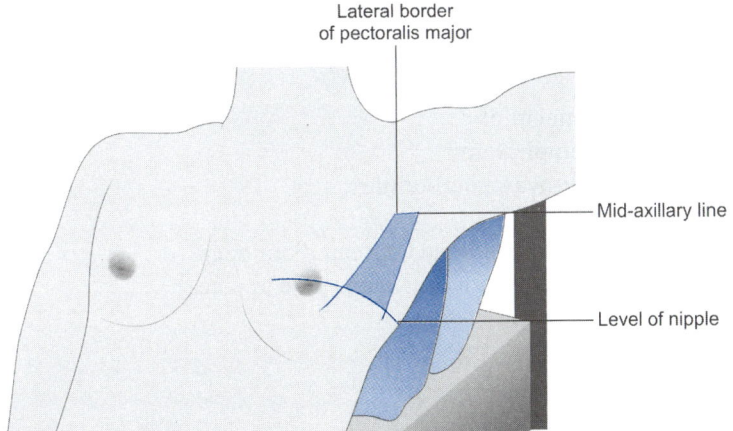

FIGURE 1.7: Safe triangle for insertion of chest tube

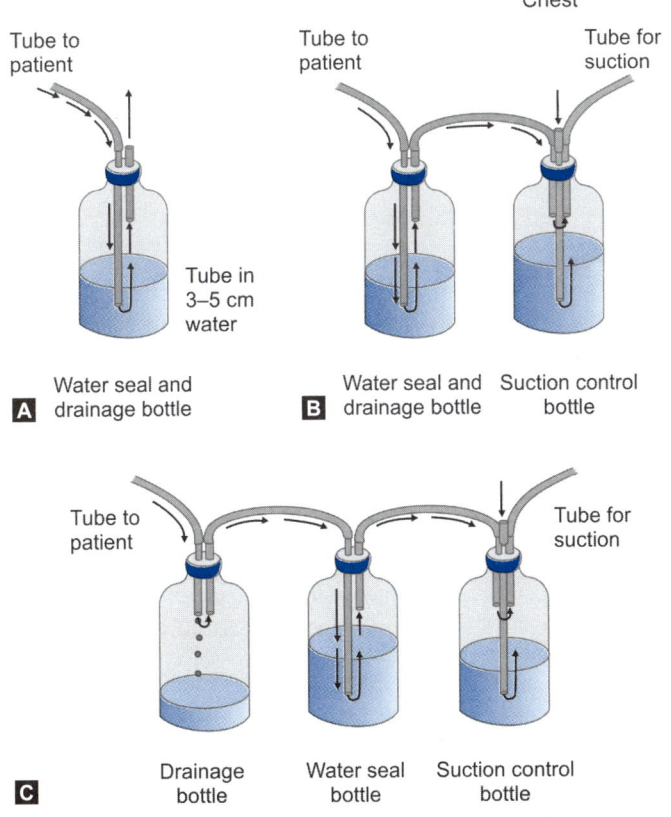

FIGURES 1.8A to C: Various types of underwater seal systems

Chest X-ray is obtained to confirm the location and also the assess lung expansion. Seldinger technique is used in selected patients and is similar to placing the central line. Caution should be exercised as the initial needle insertion can cause lung and vascular injury.

Complications

- Bleeding
- Lung parenchymal injury
- Subcutaneous emphysema
- Injury to the neurovascular bundle
- Pain
- Expansion pulmonary edema with rapid drainage
- Malposition (do not remove till a new tube in place)
- Infection.

Golden Tips

- Use ultrasound or CT scan if small effusion or possibility of difficult insertion
- Use pain relief in the form of systemic painkillers and local anesthetic
- Do not use trocar with sharp tip for insertion as it can result in parenchymal injury
- Malposition is common and new tube should be inserted prior to removal of malpositioned tube
- Limit the drainage to 1–1.5 L initially to reduce the chances of pulmonary edema.

Suggested Reading

1. American Society of Anesthesiologists Task Force on Central Venous Access (03/2012). Practice guidelies for central venous access: a report by the American Society of Anesthesiologists task force on central venous access. Anesthesiology (Philadelphia) (0003-3022), 116(3), p 539.
2. BTS guidelines for the insertion of a chest drain. Laws D, Neville E, Duffy J, on behalf of the British Thoracic Society Pleural disease group (Subgroup of the British Thoracic Society Standards of Care Committee). Thorax 2003; 58(suppl II): ii53-ii59.
3. Fishman R. Cerebrospinal fluid in diseases of the nervous system. WB Saunders. Philadelphia 1980.
4. Jubran A. Pulse oximetry. Intensive Care Med. 2004;30:2017-20.
5. Shah MR, Hasselblad V, Stevenson LW, et al. Impact of the pulmonary artery catheter in critically ill patients: meta-analysis of randomized clinical trials. JAMA. 2005; 294:1664.
6. Swan HJ, Ganz W, Forrester J, et al. Catheterization of the heart in man with use of a flow directed balloon-tipped catheter. N Engl J Med. 1970;283:447.
7. Tegtmeyer K, Brady G, Lai S, et al. Placement of an arterial line. http://content.nejm.org/cgi/video/354/15/e13 (Accessed on Feb 10, 2014).
8. www.capnography.com; Maintained by Dr Bhavani Shankar Kodali, MD. Accessed on Feb 11, 2014.

CHAPTER 2

Basic Care in ICU

Anxiety and Sedation

Anxiety and agitation is common in ICU for variety of reasons. A wide selection of medications are available to reduce this and the choice is patient dependent.

Causes of Anxiety and Distress

- Real or assumed threats by the patient of fear of treatment and treatment facilities, loss of control over situation, suffering and inability to communicate may be some of them
- Pain related to presence of endotracheal tube, tracheostomy, procedures, suctioning, therapy, trauma or surgery can all lead to pain and agitation
- Delirium (can occur in 3/4th of the patients in ICU) can be due to infection, medications, previous mental state or disorientation to the place
- Neuromuscular paralyzing agents usage for procedures or respiratory control will lead to increased use of sedative medications leading to increased agitation and confusion
- Use or withdrawal of drugs can also contribute to delirium and confusion as is common in alcohol abuse patients or drug addicts.

Presentation

- Headache, palpitations, diaphoresis, dyspnea, tachycardia, hypertension in cases of anxiety and pain issues
- Confusion, agitation, disorientation, memory loss, abnormal perception may occur in delirium and drug withdrawal
- Shallow breathing, dyspnea, hyperpnea occurs in ventilator dyssynchrony
- If able to communicate, pain scores should be used.

Treatment

Non-pharmacological Management

- Identify the cause and treat early if possible
- Try maintaining normal physiology with normal sleep cycle and lighting during the day

- Continuous orientation of the patient with family members and familiar empathetic staff helps in reducing delirium
- If on sedation, daily sedation hold with orientation
- Pain should be controlled and ventilation setting made synchronous if dyspnea present
- Medications should be checked regularly for side-effects
- Recognize drug withdrawal like alcohol and treat early
- Over sedation should be avoided and not used unless needed.

Drug Treatment

- For respiratory distress and pain, opioids like fentanyl or morphine are preferred. Painkillers like paracetamol and NSAIDs can be used as adjuncts
- For anxious patients, benzodiazepines can be used
- If delirium is present primarily, haloperidol and alpha agonists like clonidine or dexmedetomidine are preferred alongwith antipsychotics like quetiapine
- Combination of these drugs can be used depending on the etiology
- Sedative medications like propofol are added as appropriate
- Scoring systems like Richmond agitation and sedation scale (RASS) can be used to maintain the score between -2 to 0 and have been shown to reduce the length of mechanical ventilation (Table 2.1).
- Similarly for delirium in ICU, CAM-ICU (Confusion assessment method for the ICU) or similar scores can be used to initiate treatment (Table 2.2).

Table 2.1: Richmond agitation and sedation scale

Score	Descriptor	Characteristics
+4	Combative	Combative, violent, immediate danger to staff
+3	Very agitated	Pulls or removes tube(s) or catheter(s); aggressive
+2	Agitated	Frequent nonpurposeful movement, fights ventilator
+1	Restless	Anxious, apprehensive but movements not aggressive or vigorous
0	Alert and calm	
−1	Drowsy	Not fully alert, but has sustained awakening to vioce (eye opening and contact >10 seconds)
−2	Light sedation	Briefly awakens to voice (eye opening and contact <10 seconds)
−3		
−4	Moderate sedation	Movement or eye opening to voice (but no eye contact)
	Deep sedation	No response to voice, but movement or eye opening to physical stimulation
−5	Unarousable	No response to voice physical stimulation

Basic Care in ICU

Table 2.2: The confusion assessment method for the diagnosis of delirium in the ICU (CAM-ICU) (182, 185)

Feature	Assessment variables
1. Acute onset of mental status changes or Fluctuating course	Is there evidence of an acute change in mental status from the baseline? Did the (abnormal) behavior fluctuate during the past 24 hours, i.e., tend to come and go or increase and decrease in severity? Did the sedation scale (e.g., SAS or maas) or coma scale (GCS) fluctuate in the past 24 hours?
2. Inattention	Did the patient have difficulty focusing attention? How does the patient score on the Attention Screening Examination (ASE)? (i.e., Visual Component ASE tests the patient's ability to pay attention via recall of 10 pictures; auditory component ASE tests attention via having patient squeeze hannds or nod whenever the letter "A" is called in a random letter sequence)
3. Disorganized thinking	It the patient is already extubated from the ventilator, determine whether or not the patient's thinking is disorganized or incoherent, such as rambling or irrelevant conversation, unclear or illogical flow of ideas, or unpredictable switching from subject to subject. For those still on the ventilator, can the patient answer the following 4 questions correctly? 1. Will a stone float on water? 2. Are there fish in the sea? 3. Does one pound weigh more than two pounds? 4. Can you use a hammer to pound a nail? Was the patient able to follow questions and commonds throughout the assessment? 1. "Are you having any unclear thinking?" 2. "Hold up this many fingers." (examiner holds two fingers in front of patient)? 3. "Now do the same thing with the other hand." (not repeating the number of fingers)
4. Altered level of consciousness (any level of consciousness other than alert (e.g., vigilant, lethargic, stupor, or coma)	*Alert*: normal, spontaneously fully aware of environment, interacts appropriately Vigilant: hyperalert Lethargic: drowsy but easily aroused, unaware of some elements in the environment, or not spontaneously interacting appropriately with the interviewer; becomes fully aware and appropriately interactive when prodded minimally *Stuppor*: difficult to arouse, unaware of some or all elements in the environment, or not spontaneously interacting with the interviewer; becomes incompletely aware and inappropriately interactive when prodded strongly; can be aroused only by vigorous and repeated stimuli and as soon as the stimulus ceases, stuporous subjects lapse back into the unresponsive state. Coma: unarousable, unaware of all elements in the environment, with no spontaneous interaction or awareness of the interviewer, so that the interview is impossible even with maximal prodding

Patients are diagnosed with delirium if they have both Features 1 and 2 either Feature 3 or 4.
"SAS = Sedation-Analgesia Scale, MAAS = Motor Activity Assessment Scale, GCS - Glasgow Coma Scale.

CAM-ICU Scoring System

Golden Tips

- Sedation should be chosen appropriate to the patient. Oversedation should be avoided with intermittent bolus sedation preferable to continuous infusion and daily interruptions should be used whenever possible
- Scoring systems such as RASS and CAM-ICU along with are useful in assessing the agitation and initiating treatment
- Continuous orientation and maintaining good sleep-wake cycle reduces the disorientation in patients.

Depression

Depression related to the ICU admission can occur during their stay in the ICU and can continue after discharge. This can be a form of post-traumatic stress disorder requiring treatment.

Presentation

Reactive depression is common after ICU stay in many patients. The patient will be withdrawn, unhappy, hopeless, have guilt and feel worthless. There will be lack of interest in the disease and its management plans, physical activities and interest, reduced cooperation, and sometimes suicidal ideation. Many patients are not diagnosed due to other medical conditions needed more urgent attention. Post-traumatic stress disorder can be present in up to 30% of patients admitted to the ICU.

Risk Factors

- Previous history of depression
- Prolonged ICU stay
- Presence of chronic disease
- Use of benzodiazepines
- Metabolic diseases like hypothyroidism
- Lack of sleep
- Drug withdrawal including alcohol withdrawal
- History of head trauma.

Management

Regular orientation and involvement of patient and family will reduce the incidence of depression. Sleep quality should be improved and natural lighting is important. Anxiolytics are occasionally helpful in acute episodes but should not be continued indefinately. Psychiatry consult may be obtained once the patient has improved from the initial illness. Some patients will need antidepressants such as selective serotonin reuptake inhibitors (SSRIs) like paroxetine, sertraline or fluoxetine and tricyclic antidepressants like amitriptyline.

Delirium

Delirium is an acute confusional state seen commonly in the ICU population. There is altered consciousness with difficulty in focusing and attentiveness. This occurs in a short time and is fluctuating. It has to be differentiated from dementia.

Risk Factors

- Older patients
- Presence of brain diseases like dementia, Parkinsonism or stroke
- Malignancy—advanced cancer is an independent factor. This may be related to various medications given for the cancer like opioids
- Medications—opioids, psychoactive drugs, benzodiazepines
- Medical conditions—sepsis, metabolic problems, dehydration, malnutrition
- Postoperative state—due to pain, anesthetic drugs, painkillers, sedation, etc.
- Pain and painkillers—untreated pain can lead to confusion and agitation, while overuse of opioids can also lead to confusion and disorientation
- Previous drug or alcohol abuse
- Renal and hepatic impairment.

Treatment

- Recognize and treat the cause of delirium
- Check for endocrine causes
- Regular reorientation and stimulation (family can help in orientation)
- Establishing normal sleep patterns
- Correct oxygenation problems, fluid and electrolyte imbalances
- Treat sepsis aggressively and early
- Recognize drug/alcohol withdrawal and treat appropriately
- Check for medications that might be causing the delirium
- Drugs like haloperidol and clonidine can be used in severe cases, caution should be exercised with drugs and doses as most patients are elderly.

Golden Tips

- Delirium is common in elderly ICU population
- Prophylaxis is not useful in delirium
- Severe agitation may respond to haloperidol and benzodiazepines should be avoided
- Orientation and presence of family reduces the incidence of delirium.

Pain

Critically ill patients can have a lot of pain due to illness, surgical intervention, presence of tubes and lines and other procedures during their stay in the ICU. Many such patients are not able to communicate due to the presence of tubes, confusion, delirium or sedation. Pain increases the metabolic demand of the body too, so should be controlled adequately and quickly. Long-term psychiatric problems can also occur due to uncontrolled pain in ICU.

Assessment of Pain

This becomes easy if the patient is alert and orientated to the surroundings and self. Treatment can then be provided easily. Questionnaires, visual scales or other rating systems can be used for an objective measurement of pain and response to treatment. This becomes more and more difficult if the patient is sedated or confused. If grimacing or abnormal movements are present and patients exhibit sympathetic response like diaphoresis, tachypnea, tachycardia or hypertension, pain should be suspected. The behavioral pain scale or the critical care pain observation tool can also be used (Fig. 2.1).

Treatment of Pain

Painkillers that are used in ICU should have few side-effects and should act quickly without being accumulated. It is desirable to achieve a pain score of 2–3 out of 10 in ICU. Various classes of painkillers are available and used frequently in ICU.

- ❑ *Paracetamol*: It can be used in the oral form or intravenous form. Care should be taken to avoid overdose of this medication especially in the intravenous form. It also treats the pyrexia if present.
- ❑ *NSAIDs*: It can be used similarly to reduce inflammation and pyrexia. Caution should be exercised as they can lead to renal injury, bleeding in the gut and occasionally flare up bronchoconstriction. They are not as commonly used as paracetamol for this reason in ICU population.

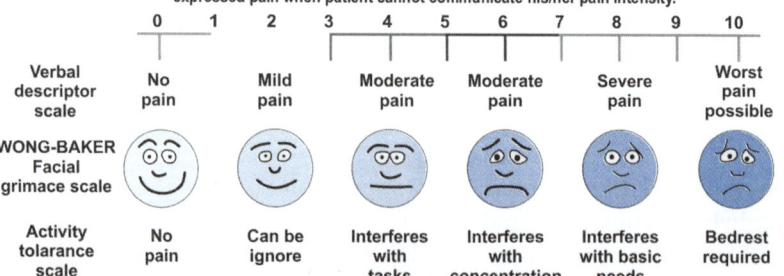

FIGURE 2.1: Universal pain assessment tool

- *Ketamine*: It is a NMDA receptor antagonist. This is occasionally used in ICU patients as an adjuvant. It has opioid sparing properties, but can lead to psychotropic effects in some patients.
- *Gabapentine*: It is a GABA analog and used in neuropathic pain. Pregabalin is another such drug.
- *Clonidine and dexmedetomidine*: These are alpha agonists with some painkilling and sedative effects. These have recently been used more in postoperative patients for fast-track extubations with some success. Clonidine can cause a drop in the blood pressure whereas dexmedetomidine is more cardiostable.
- *Opioids*: It remain the mainstay for treatment of pain in the ICU. They have a predictable and definite effect on the pain. Many drugs are available for use depending on the requirement and patient characteristics. This can range from ultra-short acting opioids like remifentanil to longer acting like diamorphine and morphine amongst others. Fentanyl and morphine are the most used opioids for pain in ICU. The side effects include sedation, respiratory depression, GI disturbances, hypotension, bradycardia and chest wall rigidity amongst others. They can also lead to tolerance and dependence occasionally. Judicious use is warranted and bolus doses preferred to infusions due to the risk of accumulation.
- Other techniques like local anesthetic infiltration, regional blocks, neuraxial techniques like epidural analgesia should be considered in all the patients to reduce the requirements of opioids and other painkillers.

Golden Tips

- Assess the pain in all the patients with visual or numeric scale and treat appropriately
- Opioids remain the mainstay for treatment of pain. Bolus doses should be preferred to continuous infusions
- Caution should be exercised especially in renal failure patients due to risk of accumulation.

Nutrition in Intensive Care Unit

Nutrition is very important for the recovery of critically-ill patients. The main aim of nutritional support is to supply necessary nutrients to meet the needs of these patients. This is more important if the patients cannot eat and drink properly on their own due to a variety of reasons.

Concepts

The initial phase of acute illness is characterized by increased metabolic demand and catabolism. Substrate utilization is altered and carbohydrates preferred to fats. Increased muscle breakdown occurs in intensive care unit

(ICU) due to inflammatory mediators and increased demand. This increases further in sepsis, burns, head injury, postoperatively and trauma. Recovery phase is an anabolic phase and during this some of the muscle repair and nutritional stores are replenished. Early nutrition will counterbalance this demand and reduce the catabolism, whereas reduced support increases loss of muscle mass, organ failure, infection, prolonged stay and mortality.

Routes for Nutrition

Enteral route of nutrition is preferred wherever possible. This reduces the incidence of infection and other complications associated with parenteral nutrition. Early enteral nutrition may reduce the incidence of infectious complications compared to late enteral nutrition. This may relate to preservation of gut immune function and reduced inflammation. Parenteral route should only be used when enteral feeding is not possible. This is because of increased infectious complications and mechanical complications associated with the parenteral route. The choice of nutrition type depends on the individual patients. Malnourished and obese patients should both have enteral nutrition if possible.

Complications

- Aspiration pneumonitis
- Diarrhea
- Refeeding syndrome (if malnourished for long time: start feeds slowly and monitor the electrolytes)
- Mechanical complications associated with insertion of nasogastric tubes and central lines for access.
- Catheter related bloodstream infections: Increased chances as total parenteral nutrition is a culture medium due to nutrients present.
- Thrombus/bleeding/embolism.

Contraindications

- Hemodynamically unstable patient on multiple inotropes/vasopressors with signs of perfusion issues
- Bowel obstruction or recent surgery
- Active GI bleed
- Parenteral nutrition is contraindicated if the patient is volume overloaded, has electrolyte imbalances and has not been tried to fed enterally.

Management

- Nutritional support should be started as soon as possible (if possible within two days of admission).
- Preference should be given to enteral nutrition over parenteral nutrition.

- If enteral route is contraindicated, parenteral nutrition should be chosen and started within a week of admission. This should be started early in case of malnourished patients with caloric deficit.
- The benefits of enteral route are reduced risk of infection, reduced electrolyte and glucose alterations, cost and regeneration of enterocytes.
- Parenteral route has the benefit of starting at any time, as it doesn't depend on gut function.
- Expert dietician support should be sought to calculate the caloric requirement along with protein, fat and carbohydrate contents of the feeds. In patients of burns, sepsis and trauma the requirements will be more, while patients who are malnourished are at risk of refeeding syndrome.
- Insulin is often needed when parenteral nutrition is started.
- If ileus present prokinetic drugs like erythromycin and metoclopramide can be tried before parenteral nutrition is started.

Requirements

- Patients weight should be taken into consideration for the calculation of nutrition requirements. For malnourished patients, their actual weight should be used; while for normal or overweight patients, their ideal weight should be used.
- Feeding can be started with 20 kcal/kg/day calorie diet and increased appropriately depending on the demand and state of patient.
- Protein requirements are around 0.8-1.2 g/kg/day but many patients especially burns patients may require up to 2g/kg/day.
- Lipids and electrolytes are added to the above regime as required.

Golden Tips

- Enteral route should be preferred as far as possible and started early
- If patients are unstable and on multiple inotropes/vasopressors, consider reducing or stopping enteral feeds.
- Aggressive feeding in a malnourished patient may lead to fluid and electrolyte abnormalities (refeeding syndrome).

Blood Sugar Control in ICU

Raised glucose levels in intensive care unit (ICU) can be due to many reasons including previous history of diabetes, stress response (cortisol, catecholamines, glucagon), drugs (steroids, catacholamines, parenteral nutrition) and insulin resistance. Poor control can lead to increased morbidity and mortality.

Concepts

Hyperglycemia is associated with worse outcomes in multiple group of ICU patients including trauma, medical and surgical patients. This may be related to its effect on white cell function, increased risk of infection, cardiac effects, polymyoneuropathy—all leading to increased morbidity and length of stay in the hospital. It is accepted now that hyperglycemia should be controlled, but the actual level of blood sugar control remains controversial. Strict control (80–110 mg/dL) may be beneficial but leads to increased risk of hypoglycemia. Meta-analysis of the trials supports a less stringent control of blood sugar to avoid hypoglycemia and mortality in the intensive control group. Most centers would now prefer a glucose target range between 140–180 mg/dL. This avoids hypoglycemia episodes and the morbidity associated with it.

Methods of Glucose Control

Various methods of glucose control are used in the ICU. The best approach would be to start an insulin infusion in acutely ill patients with regular monitoring of blood glucose levels. This is because of poor absorption from subcutaneous tissue and rapid changes in intrinsic catecholamine/hormone levels and use of extrinsic drugs. Once the glucose is controlled and the acute situation improves, this can be transitioned to sliding scale insulin subcutaneously and then longer acting insulin depending on the nutrition and glucose levels. Oral drugs can then be established in consultation with the endocrinologists.

Golden Tips

- Target the blood glucose between 140–180 mg/dL compared to the strict target of 80–110 mg/dL
- Preferably use the insulin infusion to start with in an acutely sick patient, slowly transitioning to sliding scale or long acting insulin
- Regular blood glucose measurements should be done for better control of blood glucose.

Prevention of Gastric Ulcer in ICU

Stress ulcers in intensive care unit (ICU) patients generally occur in the body or fundus of the stomach. They are generally shallow with superficial oozing, but deep lesions may occur occasionally leading to catastrophic bleeding. Erosions may be present in up to 20% of ICU patients, but bleeding can occur in up to 10% patients. Severe complications are rare (up to 1% patients).

Causes and Risks

Stress ulcers can be caused due to impaired defence mechanism or increased acid secretions. Multiple physiological derangements may lead to the above including impaired perfusion, uremia and other toxins; head injury per se may increase the acid secretion. The presence of *Helicobacter pylori* infection may also contribute as defence mechanisms are compromised.

Basic Care in ICU

Risk factors for development of GI bleed are:
- Coagulopathy
- Head or spinal trauma
- Mechanical ventilation
- Hepatic or renal failure
- Coagulopathy
- Previous history of peptic ulcer disease or upper GI bleed
- Multiple trauma
- Shock/sepsis
- Burns
- Steroid/NSAID/aspirin use.

The presence of GI bleeding increases the morbidity and mortality in ICU patients.

Ulcer Prophylaxis

Ulcer prophylaxis should be used in ICU patients with any of the major or 2 or more minor criteria:

Major

- Mechanical ventilation for >2 days
- History of GI bleed or ulcer in past 1 year
- Coagulopathy.

Minor

- Sepsis
- ICU admission lasting >1 week
- Occult GI bleed >5 days
- Glucocorticoid therapy.

This should also be considered in major burns patients and patients with head injury or spinal injury. Patients on enteral feed have reduced risk of ulceration and hence this is not routinely recommended.

Commonly used Agents

- *H2 blockers*: They reduce the gastric acid secretion by acting on the H2 receptors on parietal cell. Oral and intravenous formulations are available. Ranitidine is the most commonly used drug in this class
- *Proton-pump inhibitors*: They block the acid secretion by inhibiting the H-K pump. Oral and intravenous formulations are available and omeprazole is the commonly used agent
- *Sucralfate*: this coats and protects the mucosa, without altering the pH and secretion. This can be given 1g four times a day. Small risk of aluminium toxicity exists but is not commonly seen. Also its higher volume and granularity may preclude its use.

- *Antacids*: Similar use as sucralfate. Difficulty in administration through nasogastric (NG) tube.
- *Others*: Misoprostal has been used in NSAID induced ulceration. Limited data on use and safety.

Data suggests that proton pump-inhibitor (PPI) have a lower rate of bleeding compared to H2 blockers; which in turn has a lower rate compared to antacids and sucralfate. Small risk of increase in pneumonia exists with pH lowering medications though. Overall PPIs and H2 blockers are recommended for ICU patiens with a case by case selection of the agent.

Golden Tips

- Ulcer prophylaxis should be used if any major or 2 or more minor criteria are present in ICU patients
- H2 blockers or PPI are both effective but may increase the incidence of pneumonia
- Patients on full enteral feeds do not need ulcer prophylaxis generally
- Prophylaxis should be discontinued when possible as the risk reduction is minimal in normal patients.

Thromboprophylaxis in ICU

Venous thromboembolism (VTE) remains the most common preventable cause of morbidity and mortality in the hospitals. The difference in outcomes exists between surgical and medical patients; with surgical patients benefiting with use of thromboprophylaxis more than the medical patients. This may be due to the difference in coexisting and complex medical problems in medical patients. There has been a massive drive to consider thromboprophylaxis in all hospital patients to reduce the risk of venous thromboembolism.

Risk Factors for Developing VTE

- *Hospitalization*: This increases the risk due to the medical condition, reduced mobility and medications
- *ICU stay*: This increases the risk further. Even with the used of prophylaxis, the incidence remains high
- *Pregnancy*: It is a hypercoagulable state. The incidence is more common in patients having cesarian section in the postoperative period
- Obesity
- Previous VTE
- Inherited or acquired prothrombotic state
- Cancer
- Immobility
- Presence of invasive lines.

The above combined with release of prothrombotic cytokines, stasis and stress hormone release increases the risk of VTE. Surgical patients have a hypercoaguable state leading to VTE with an even higher chance in patients with long bone fractures.

Risk Assessment

Various scoring systems can be used for selecting the appropriate patients for prophylaxis. For medical patients, this includes IMPROVE and Padua Prediction Score. In surgical patients, Caprini score is used most commonly. IMPROVE score uses the following criteria to define the estimated risk of acute symptomatic VTE:
- Previous VTE (risk of 3.1%)
- Thrombophilia (risk of 3.1%)
- Current cancer (risk of 1%)
- Age more than 60 years (risk of 1%).

If there is presence of more than one factors, the risk will be synergistic. Caprini score uses age, type and severity of surgical insult, obesity, vasculopathy, presence of sepsis or lung disease, trauma, malignancy, limb surgery or fracture, etc. to calculate a score. The therapy is then started depending on the score calculated.

Prophylaxis and Prevention

Primary prophylaxis will depend on individual risk of VTE. Drugs and mechanical methods are used to prevent DVT. Secondary prevention is used to detect and treat developed DVT and PE in a patient. Caution should be exercised and risk-benefit assessed in patients who are at high-risk of bleeding.
- Ambulation of the patient as early as possible will reduce the incidence of VTEs. This is enough for very low-risk patients
- Mechanical methods should be used in everyone admitted to the hospital unless there are contraindications. This includes use of graduated compression stockings and sequential compression devices. This is used in all patients with more than very low-risk and also in patients where medications are contraindicated. Caution should be exercised in patients with varicose veins or vasculopathy as this may hamper the blood supply to the limbs
- Moderate to high-risk patients should all have pharmacological prophylaxis. The drugs commonly used include:
  - *Low molecular weight heparin*: This is the most common drug used for prophylaxis. Depending on the weight and indication this can be given once or twice a day and doesn't need monitoring. Various drugs are available including enoxaparin, tinzaparin.
  - *Unfractionated heparin*: Due to shorter half life, this needs to be given 2–3 times a day. It is useful if a patient has renal dysfunction and can be monitored easily with INR. It is less efficacious compared to LMWHs.

- *Fondaparinux*: This can be used in patients reacting to heparins. This can be given once a day again and is sometimes preferred if concomitant ischaemic heart disease exists.
- *Warfarin*: Warfarin is used when long-term anticoagulation is warranted because of either pre-existing use or presence of DVT/PE.
- *Others*: Drugs like aspirin are not useful for prophylaxis, though can be used if other drugs are contraindicated. Other direct thrombin and factor Xa inhibitors (rivaroxaban) are being studied in selected patients.
- *Inferior vena cava filter*: This has been used in patients with high-risk of DVT/presence of DVT, where thromboprophylaxis is contraindicated.

Golden Tips

- All patients admitted to the hospital or ICU should be assessed for the need of thromboprophylaxis using one of the scoring systems
- Low molecular weight heparins are preferred due to better efficacy, single daily (or twice daily) dosing and absence of need for monitoring
- In renal failure, unfractionated heparin should be used
- Mechanical methods should be used in all patients unless contraindicated.

Suggested Reading

1. Barr J, Fraser G, Puntillo K, et al. Clinical practice guidelines for the management of pain, agitation and delirium in adult patients in the intensive care unit. Critical Care Med. 2013;41(1):263-306.
2. Caprini JA. Thrombosis risk assessment as a guide to quality patient care. Dis Mon. 2005;51(2-3):70-8.
3. Davydow DS, Gifford JM, Desai SV, Bienvenu OJ, Needham DM. Depression in general intensive care unit survivors: a systemic review. Intensive Care Med. 2009;35:796-809.
4. Guillamondegui OD, Gunter OL, Bonadies JA, et al. Practice management guidelines for stress ulcer prophylaxis. Eastern Association for the Surgery of Trauma (EAST), Chicago. 2008. Pp. 1-24.
5. http://www.outcomesumassmed.org/IMPROVE/risk_score/vte/index.html. Accessed on 15th Feb, 2014.
6. McClave SA, Martindale RG, Vanek VW, et al. Guidelines for the provision and assessment of nutrition support therapy in the adult critically ill patient: Society of Critical Care Medicine (SCCM) and American Society for Parenteral and enteral nutrition (ASPEN). J Parenter Enteral Nutr. 2009;33(3):277-316.
7. Mularski RA. Pain management in the intensive care unit. Crit Care Clin. 2004;20(3):381-401.
8. Pisani MA, McNicoll L, Inouye SK. Cognitive impairment in the intensive care unit. Clin Chest Med. 2003;24(4):727-37.
9. The NICE-SUGAR Study Investigators. Hypoglycemia and risk of death in critically ill patients. N Engl J Med. 2012;367:1108-18.
10. Van den Berghe G, Wouters P, Weekers F, et al. Intensive insulin therapy in critically ill patients. N Engl J Med. 2001;345(19):1359-67.

CHAPTER 3

Cardiovascular System

Stable Angina Pectoris

Presentation and Diagnosis

Angina pectoris or angina is chest pain arising due to ischemia of heart muscle related to either increased demand or reduced supply of oxygen to the muscle. Stable angina presents as a sub-sternal heaviness and discomfort induced by anxiety or exertion, lasting few minutes and relieved by rest or GTN spray. This may radiate to the arms or jaw and have nausea/vomiting or shortness of breath associated. ECG may be normal or show ST-T changes that is normalized on taking rest. Stress testing with exercise or drugs and angiography will confirm the suspicion.

Risk Factors

- Age >55 for men and >65 for women
- Cigarette smoking
- Diabetes
- Hypertension
- Family history
- Dyslipidemia
- Renal impairment
- Obesity
- Stress
- Drugs like cocaine
- Severe anemia.

Differential Diagnosis

- Unstable angina
- Pericarditis
- Musculoskeletal pain
- Dissection
- Gastroesophageal reflux
- Pulmonary embolism
- Peptic ulcer disease.

Management

Pain relief with opioids, aspirin, supplemental oxygen if needed, nitrates for symptom relief. This can then be supplemented with beta-blockers and calcium channel blockers along with advice on lifestyle modifications, statin and blood pressure control.

Unstable Angina

Presentation and Diagnosis

Similar presentation as stable angina; but diagnosed as unstable if:
- Increasing frequency or duration of angina
- Poor relief with GTN spray
- Angina at rest or minimal exertion
- New onset or severe pain
- Dynamic changes in the ECG.

It is termed as non-ST segment elevation myocardial infarction, if it is associated with enzyme elevation (cardiac troponins) suggesting muscle damage. If it is occurring at rest, it portends a worse prognosis as it may be a serious indicator of subsequent myocardial infarction. It usually occurs due to platelet aggregation on normal endothelium, coronary artery spasms or coronary thrombosis. Most such attacks occur in the night-time at rest.

Differential diagnosis is similar to angina pectoris.

Management

Initial treatment as stable angina pectoris. Serial ECG and enzyme levels should be done. Treatment includes aspirin, statins, beta-blockers and nitrates for symptoms. Consider ACE-inhibitors if diabetic or evidence of heart failure. Clopidogrel is used and crescendo attacks should be treated with anticoagulation with heparin/low molecular weight heparin. Further interventions like angiography and angioplasty should be considered under the cover of clopidogrel and heparin/low molecular weight heparin. If percutaneous intervention is considered, GPIIb/IIIa inhibitors should be considered.

Myocardial Infarction (ST Segment Elevation)

Presentation and Diagnosis

This presents as a prolonged chest pain, which might be very similar to stable, or unstable angina, but usually lasting more than 15 minutes. This might be associated with hypotension and cardiac failure or sudden onset of arrhythmias. ECG is typified with ST segment elevation or more than 1 mm in two contiguous leads or new onset LBBB (Figs 3.1 and 3.2). Elevation of cardiac

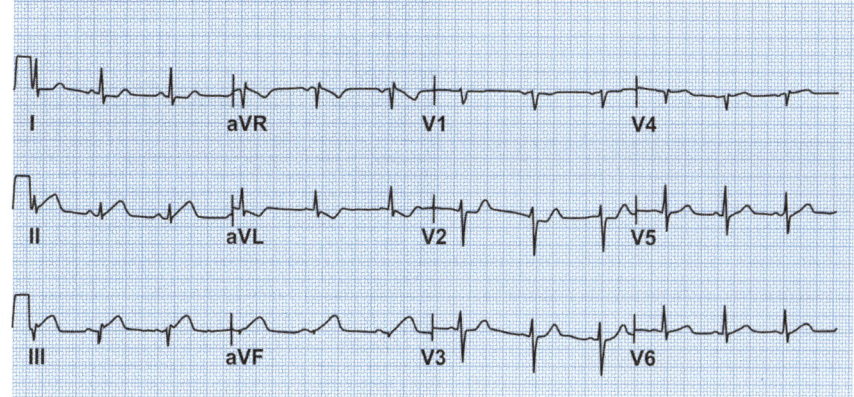

FIGURE 3.1: ECG showing inferior wall myocardial infarction (II/III/aVF)

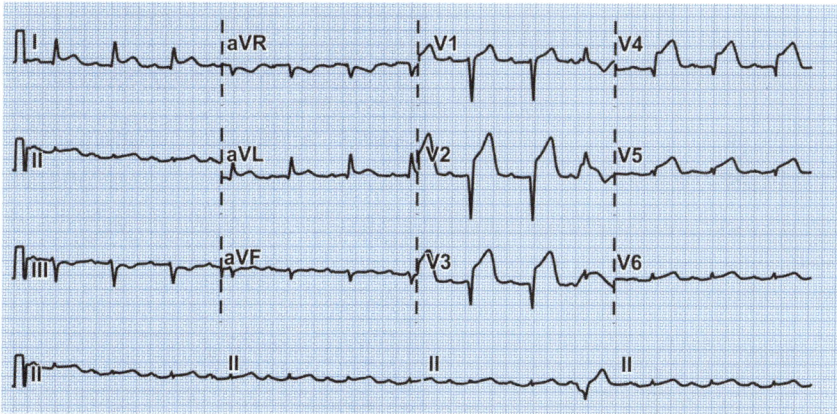

FIGURE 3.2: ECG showing anterior wall myocardial infarction (V1-V5)

enzymes is seen and ECHO if done during the episode will suggest wall motion abnormalities in the suspected area. This can be complicated with arrhythmia, cardiac failure, and wall or papillary rupture.

The differential diagnosis is similar to stable or unstable angina.

Management

Rest, oxygen if needed, pain relief and ECGs are essential. Aspirin is given immediately. Beta-blockers can reduce myocardial demand and ACE-inhibitors are given if tolerated in suspicion of cardiac failure.

Once the diagnosis and territory of infarct is clear, primary angioplasty has better results in the long and short-terms. If resources for this are not available, thrombolysis with drugs is second option. If the patient continues to have angina like symptoms after thrombolysis, a secondary angioplasty can be done to improve symptoms. The precipitating factors should be investigated and life-style modifications should be explained to the patients. Aspirin, beta-blockers and ACE-inhibitors should be considered along with statins in all patients. Patients with reduced cardiac function will benefit from ACE-inhibitors and spironolactone to prevent ventricular wall remodeling.

Bradycardia and Heart Block

Types and Causes

Heart rate of less than 60 per minute is considered as bradycardia. This is common in athletes and young people, patients on drugs like beta-blockers, digoxin and non-dihydropyridine calcium channel blockers. If asymptomatic, no treatment is necessary.

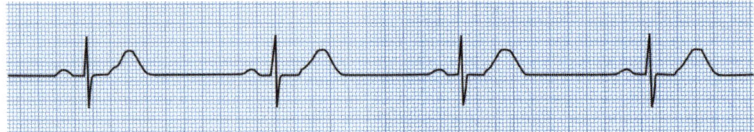

FIGURE 3.3: Sinus bradycardia

First Degree AV Block

Heart blocks are generally as a result of conduction problems through the AV node. First-degree heart block is a prolonged PR interval suggesting delay in AV conduction.

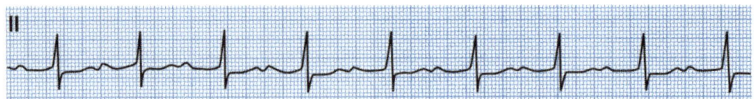

FIGURE 3.4: First degree AV block (increased PR interval)

Second Degree AV Block

Second-degree heart block is of two types:
 a. Mobitz type 1 (Wenckebach's phenomenon) is a result of sequential prolongation of PR interval followed by a missed conduction. Both first degree and mobitz type 1 blocks are seen in people with increased vagal tone (athletes/drugs/young people) and are generally asymptomatic and don't warrant treatment.

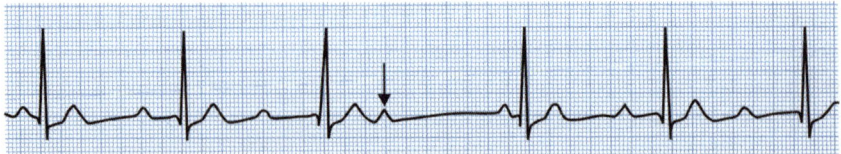

FIGURE 3.5: Mobitz type 1 AV block

b. Mobitz type 2 block is intermittent blocked beats without a change in PR intervals.

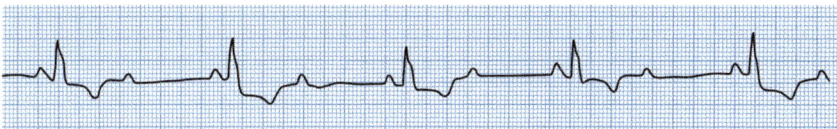

FIGURE 3.6: Mobitz type 2 AV block

Third Degree AV Block

Third degree heart block has complete AV dissociation. Both Mobitz type 2 and third degree heart blocks suggest cardiac problems and warrant further management. These can be associated with symptoms of cardiac failure and angina, electrolyte abnormalities, etc.

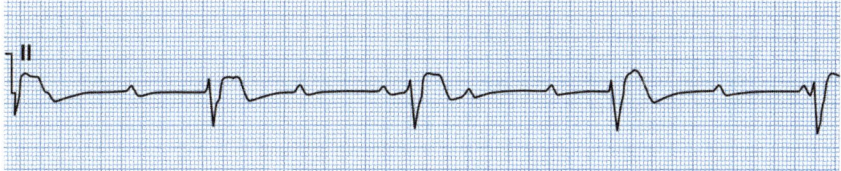

FIGURE 3.7: Third degree AV block

Management

Management depends on the stability of the patient. Oxygen therapy should be started if unstable or low saturations are present. Vagolytics like atropine can be used to stabilize initially. A dose of more than 0.5 mg is generally used to prevent reactive bradycardia. Isoprenaline or other beta-agonists like adrenaline or dopamine can also be useful as temporary measures. Temporary pacemaker should be set-up, which can be transcutaneous, or transvenous; followed by permanent pacemaker insertion if the cause is irreversible. Drugs that can cause heart blocks should be stopped and electrolytes corrected.

Atrial Fibrillation

Causes and Diagnosis

This is characterized by irregularly irregular ventricular response to a chaotic atrial activity. The irregularity usually originates from the roots of the pulmonary veins. ECG shows absence of P waves and irregularly irregular ventricular response.

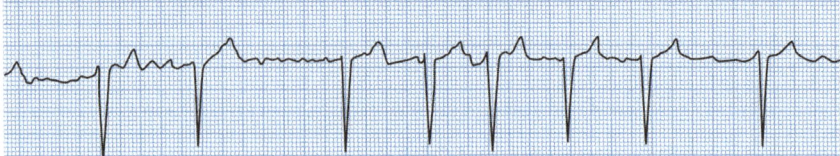

FIGURE 3.8: ECG showing atrial fibrillation

Atrial Fibrillation with Fibrillatory Waves

This can be associated with symptoms of angina, cardiac failure, poor peripheral perfusion or thromboembolic events.

Differential Diagnosis

- Atrial flutter with variable block
- Multifocal atrial tachycardia
- Sinus arrhythmia
- Existence of pre-excitatory pathways.

This rhythm is always abnormal and can result due to ischemic heart disease, valvular heart disease, electrolyte abnormalities, heart surgeries, thyroid disorders, sepsis, and alcohol intake. This is one of the most common arrhythmia encountered in intensive care.

Management

Once atrial fibrillation is diagnosed, it should be determined if this is causing any hemodynamic compromise or not. Look for the cause with blood tests and echocardiogram. In case of compromise, electrical cardioversion can be attempted after heparin anticoagulation. If the onset is >2 days, anticoagulation should be undertaken as the risk of thromboembolism is higher. In acute situations, the cardioversion is carried out after a negative echocardiogram; but otherwise 4 weeks wait is required after starting anticoagulation. If there is no compromise, it should be determined if this is new onset or old. Fluid and electrolyte imbalances should be corrected especially potassium and magnesium levels. Most of the chronic fibrillations would not revert back to sinus rhythm. These cases should have rate controlled with drugs such as beta-blockers, calcium-channel blockers or digoxin based on their cardiac function. Amiodarone is used for pharmacological cardioversion and rate control if there is no hemodynamic compromise. Anticoagulation should be maintained with either heparin or warfarin. The following algorithm can be used to treat atrial fibrillation (Flowchart 3.1).

Cardiovascular System 35

Flowchart 3.1: Algorithm for treatment of atrial fibrillation

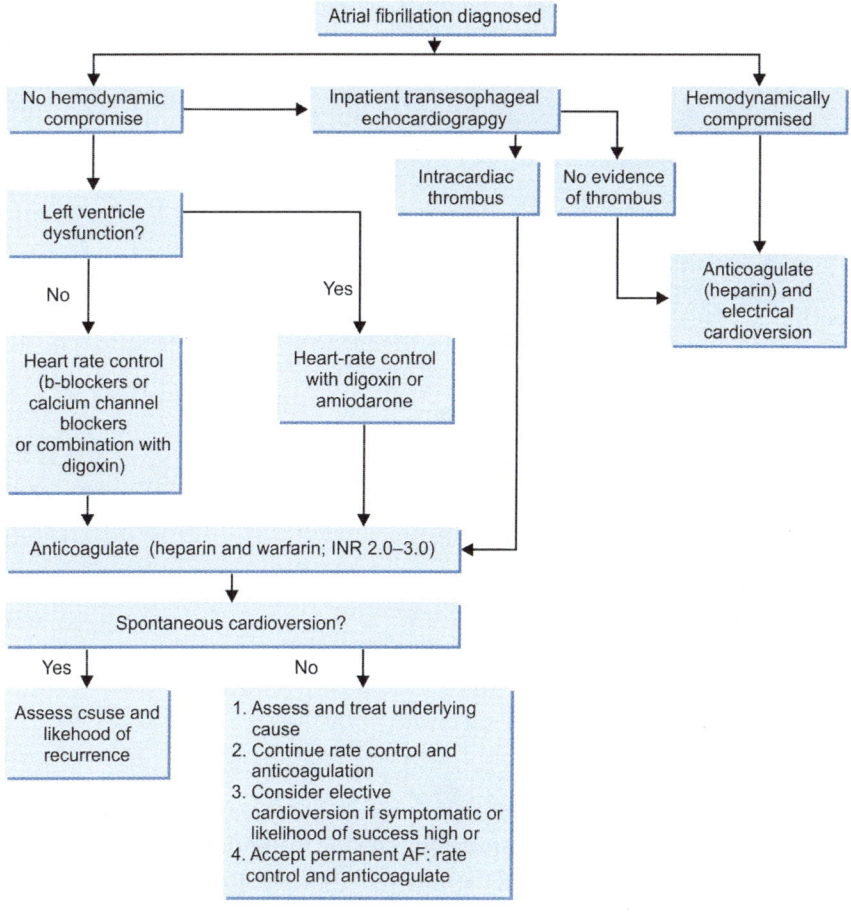

Supraventricular Tachycardia

Diagnosis and Differentials

This is tachycardia that originates from the atria or AV node. The QRS complexes are usually narrow and regular and the rate is around 150–180 per minutes. This should be differentiated from the more dangerous ventricular tachycardia. SVT is not life-threatening, but can cause symptoms and worsen heart function if not treated. The symptoms are palpitations and occasionally angina and signs of heart failure. Two common types are seen:
- Atrioventricular reciprocating tachycardia
- AV nodal re-entrant tachycardia.

Atrial fibrillation is another type of supraventricular tachycardia, but is discussed separately.

The ECG is generally diagnostic. The QRS complexes are narrow, but can be wide when there is aberrancy in conduction and has to then be differentiated from ventricular tachycardia. If the rate is even higher, accessory tract may be present along with delta waves.

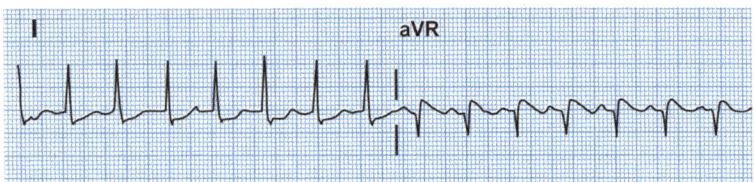

FIGURE 3.9: ECG showing supraventricular tachycardia

Supraventricular Tachycardia

Differential Diagnosis

- Sinus tachycardia
- Atrial flutter
- Atrial fibrillation
- Multifocal atrial tachycardia
- Ventricular tachycardia (differentiate from aberrant conduction in SVT)
- Junctional tachycardia.

Management

The SVT can be unpleasant, though is rarely life threatening. If AV node is involved in the increased transmission, slowing the node can revert the sinus rhythm. Otherwise the slowing may demonstrate the underlying rhythm.
- Physical maneuvers:
  - Vagal nerve activation can be carried out by asking patient to hold his breath, coughing, cold water or carotid sinus massage.
- Medications:
  - Adenosine is an ultra-short acting AV node blocking agent. This is used to terminate or show the underlying rhythm
  - Verapamil or diltiazem (calcium channel blockers) can be used if unsuccessful with adenosine or for long-term treatment
  - Beta-blockers like metoprolol can be used if the above fail and also in cases where coronary artery disease is implicated
  - If AV node is not involved, drugs like sotalol or amiodarone can be tried.
- Electrical cardioversion:
  - This is used when the patient is unstable or other treatments have not been effective. Lower Joules are used as this is sensitive to low energy.
  - Overdrive pacing can be tried if the drugs fail to convert the rhythm.
  - Electrophysiological studies are warranted in refractory cases.

Ventricular Tachycardia

Diagnosis

It is defined as presence of 3 or more consecutive ventricular beats (broad QRS complexes) at a rate of more than 100 per minute. This is a potentially life threatening arrhythmia and can deteriorate into ventricular fibrillation, asystole and sudden death. It is non-sustained if lasts <30 seconds and sustained if more than that. ECG is key to diagnosis.

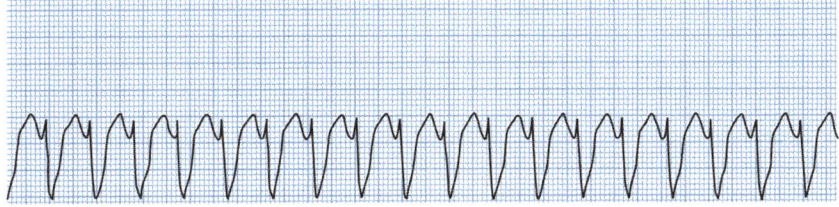

FIGURE 3.10: ECG showing ventricular tachycardia

Ventricular Tachycardia

The signs and symptoms of this arrhythmia can be:
- Heart failure
- Angina
- Palpitations
- Syncope
- Sudden death.

VT can be monomorphic or polymorphic: The later is seen in torsades de pointes (twisting of points), which can degenerate, into ventricular fibrillation (pre-morbid rhythm).

VT can be a result of ischemic heart disease, valvular heart disease, electrolyte imbalances, drug toxicity, and cardiac surgery. It is differentiated from supraventricular tachycardia (with aberrant conduction) with presence of AV dissociation, extreme axis deviation, failure of adenosine, and QRS concordance.

Management

Cardioversion is preferred if haemodynamically compromised ventricular tachycardia or fibrillation is present. Adenosine can be tried if high suspicion of supraventricular tachycardia to diagnose the underlying rhythm. If the patient is hemodynamically stable, chemical cardioversion can be tried with amiodarone. Other drugs like lignocaine, flecainide or procainamide can also be tried. Magnesium is the treatment of choice in torsades de pointes. Cardiac ablation can be tried in recurrent VT patients with difficulty in medical treatment.

Mitral Valve

Diagnosis

Mitral valve is affected very commonly and mitral regurgitation remains the most common valvular heart disease. Mitral stenosis commonly occurs in patients with rheumatic heart disease and both can coexist in these cases. Various murmurs associated with valvular diseases are shown in Figure 3.11.

Mitral Stenosis

This commonly presents with dyspnea, orthopnea, cough and rarely hemoptysis. These can vary depending upon the rapidity of onset of the lesions. The diagnosis is based on the echocardiography. On auscultation, mitral stenosis has a diastolic low-pitched murmur following an opening snap and a loud S1. There is usually atrial fibrillation associated due to enlargement of the left atrium and more common in rheumatic heart disease patients.

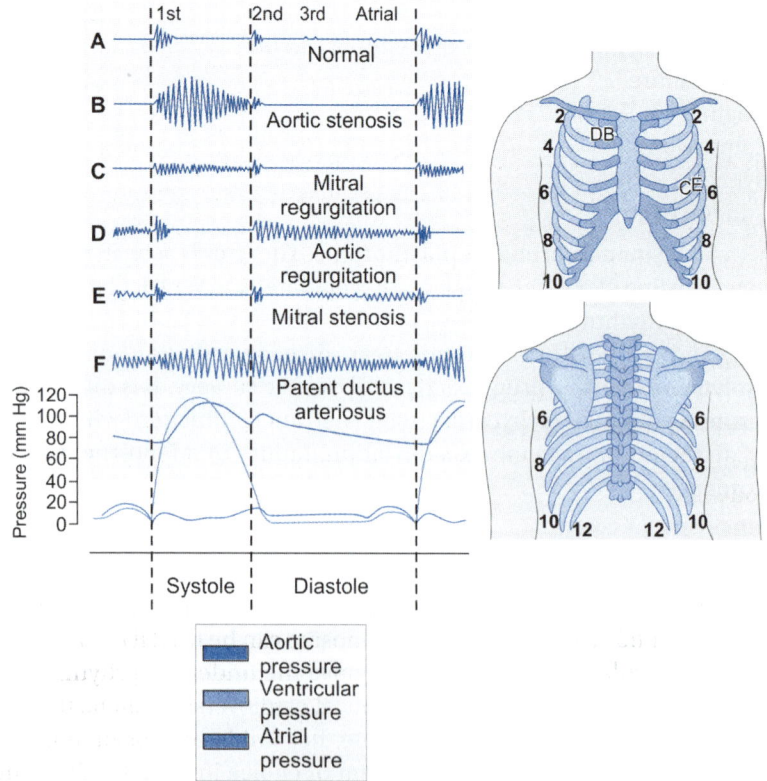

FIGURE 3.11: Phonocardiograms from normal and abnormal heart sounds
Source: Madhero88 (Own work)

Cardiovascular System

Differential Diagnosis

- Atrial myxoma
- Mitral valve prolapse
- Atrial septal defect.

Mitral Regurgitation

MR presents with a pan-systolic murmur and can be due to rheumatic heart disease, left ventricular failure, endocarditis, Marfan's syndrome, papillary muscle rupture due to myocardial infarction/ischemic heart disease. This is the most common valvular heart disease. The symptoms are congestive cardiac failure, palpitations, cardiogenic shock (in acute MR). CXR will show enlarged cardiac silhouette, ECG will have P mitrale and possible atrial fibrillation, but echocardiography is diagnostic.

Differential Diagnosis

- Hypertrophic cardiomyopathy
- Ventricular septal defect
- Tricuspid regurgitation
- Aortic stenosis.

Management

In mitral stenosis, slowing of heart rate will increase ventricular filling especially with atrial fibrillation. Cardioversion can be attempted, but large atrial size makes it more difficult. Rate control can be achieved with beta-blockers, digoxin or calcium channel blockers. Diuretics can be used to reduce pulmonary edema. Digoxin and anticoagulation are used in cases of atrial fibrillation patients. Balloon valvoplasty and valve replacements should be considered.

In mitral regurgitation, afterload reduction and heart rate at the higher end of normal to increase forward flow improves symptoms. Acute MR may need urgent surgery if there is rupture of chordae tendinae. Vasodilators can be used in the interim (nitroprusside) to decrease the regurgitant fraction if hemodynamically stable. In chornic MR, drugs like ACE- inhibitors, nitrates, diuretics and hydrallazine can be tried. Digoxin and antiarrhythmics are used in patients with atrial fibrillation. Mitral valve replacement or repair is considered in selective cases. Infective endocarditis prophylaxis should be considered as per guidance.

Aortic Valve

Diagnosis

Aortic valve disease is again classified into aortic stenosis and regurgitation. Aortic stenosis remains the most common valvular disease in the western world.

Aortic stenosis is narrowing of the aortic valve leading to increased flow velocity through the valve during systole. It presents with dyspnea, cough, syncopal episodes, angina or orthopnea related to the decreased cardiac output resulting from this. There may be associated angiodysplasia of the colon (Heyde's syndrome) and acquired von Willebrand disease. On examination the pulse pressure will be low and a harsh crescendo-decrescendo systolic murmur will be present. There is associated ventricular hypertrophy related to increased effort of the heart to pump blood across a stenosed valve. ECG will show left ventricular strain pattern and occasional conduction defects, while echocardiogram is diagnostic. CXR may demonstrate calcified aorta and in chronic cases left ventricular dilatation. The common causes for aortic stenosis are bicuspid valve, rheumatic disease and senile calcification.

Aortic regurgitation presents with heart failure and shows a widened pulse pressure and various signs associated with it (Quincke's pulse, Duroziez sign, water hammer pulse). This can result from rheumatic heart disease, endocarditis, and rarely from syphilis, aortic dissection, bicuspid valve, etc. Echocardiography as in mitral disease is essential for diagnosis.

Management

Medical management is of limited value in aortic stenosis. ACE-inhibitors and bisphosphonates have been implicated in slowing the disease, but not confirmed. Beta blockers and calcium channel blockers are used in angina symptoms. Surgery is the mainstay of treatment with valve replacement although valvoplasty can be tried in the interim. Apicoaortic conduit, percutaneous valve replacement and balloon valvuloplasty have all been tried with success.

In aortic regurgitation, afterload reduction and a mild increase in heart rate increases the forward flow. Diuretics, ACE inhibitors, and nitrates can be used. In cases of heart failure or rheumatic heart disease, digoxin is of value. Infective endocarditis prophylaxis should be considered in all cases.

Cardiac Tamponade

Presentation and Diagnosis

Cardiac tamponade occurs on a background of pericardial effusion when there is associated hemodynamic compromise with it. This occurs when the effusion starts pressing on the heart muscle leading to this compromise. It this occurs slowly, it is tolerated well with the expansion of the pericardial sac; but if it occurs rapidly, a small amount of fluid can lead to compromise. Cardiac tamponade can rarely present as a triad of hypotension, increased JVP and muffled heart sounds (Beck's triad). More than likely it will have one or two of these features. Tachycardia, pulsus paradoxus, dyspnea, palpitations and poor peripheral perfusion are more common. Chest X-ray may demonstrate enlarged cardiac shadow, but the symptoms relate to the rapidity of fluid

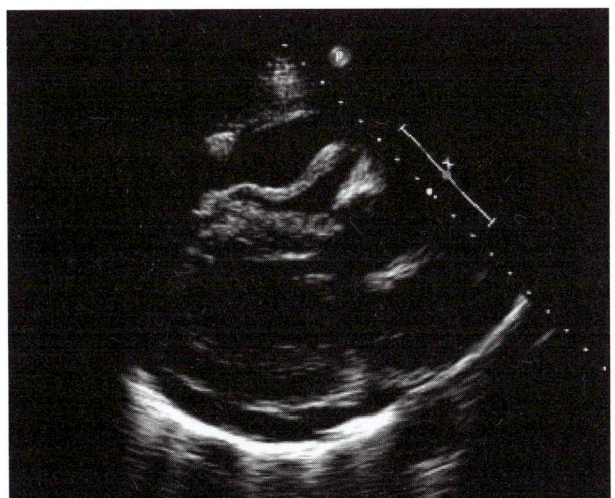

FIGURE 3.12: Cardiac tamponade on echocardiogram

collection. ECG may show tachycardia and low voltages. ECHO is paramount in diagnosis and will show fluid around the heart. It might also demonstrate the swinging of heart in the fluid in cases of large effusions, and diastolic collapse of the right heart (Fig. 3.12).

Causes

- Pericarditis
- Malignancy
- Infections
- Ventricular rupture
- Aortic dissection
- Trauma
- Postoperatively
- Uremia.

Differential Diagnosis

- Acute severe asthma
- Constrictive pericarditis
- Pneumothorax
- Restrictive cardiomyopathy.

Management

Look for the underlying cause and treat the cause to prevent further accumulation of fluid. If hemodynamic compromise is present, echocardiography followed by expert opinion on possibility of drainage of effusion should be sought. Fluid challenge followed by inotropes can be used in the interim. In chronic cases a surgical window may be tried.

Congestive Cardiac Failure

Diagnosis

Congestive cardiac (heart) failure occurs when the heart is not able to pump enough blood based on body's requirements. This can lead to shortness of breath, leg swelling, paroxysmal nocturnal dyspnea, weight gain, orthopnea and reduced exercise tolerance. Examination will reveal raised JVP, crackles in the chest, hepatomegaly, gallop rhythm, leg swelling, ascites or generalized anasarca. CXR will reveals cardiomegaly, pulmonary edema (upper lobe diversion of vasculature/bat wing appearance) and pleural effusions. There may be presence of hypoxia and bloods may reveal the cause of the cardiac failure and show increased B natriuretic peptide. Echo will reveal reduced ejection fraction or diastolic filling problem.

Types

- *Left heart failure*: This will present with pulmonary symptoms with shortness of breath, pulmonary rales, effusions and in severe cases cyanosis. There might be presence of 3rd heart sounds, paroxysmal nocturnal dyspnea, orthopnea and fatigue. Wheezing may be seen in some cases and evidence of end organ damage will begin.
- *Right heart failure*: This presents with systemic symptoms of leg edema, liver congestion, ascites and generalized anasarca. There is weight gain and nocturia in these patients.

Causes

- Myocardial infarction
- Coronary artery disease
- Hypertensive cardiac disease
- Diabetes
- Valvular heart disease
- Cardiomyopathy
- Toxins and alcohol.

Differential Diagnosis

- ARDS
- Fluid overload
- Protein deficiency (malnourishment)
- Valvular heart disease
- Thyroid disorders.

Management

In acute distress, oxygen with pre- and after-load reductions are achieved with diuretics, nitrates, and morphine. Non-invasive ventilation may be required to reduce pulmonary edema. In chronic cases, ACE inhibitors or angiotensin receptor blockers are used if tolerated along with spironolactone to reduce mortality from cardiac failure. Beta-blockers should be used whenever tolerated to reduce long-term mortality. Digoxin is proven to reduce morbidity and hospital admissions. Salt reduction and physical activity as tolerated should be recommended. Blood pressure control is important in diastolic heart failure. Surgery is considered in selective cases with heart transplant, and left ventricular assist device. As a bridge to surgery various inotropes and intra-aortic balloon pump may be tried.

Aortic Dissection

Presentation

Aortic dissection occurs when a tear in the inner wall of aorta leads to blood collection between layers of its wall. This presents as a severe tearing chest pain that might radiate to the back. This may be associated with weakness or paraplegia, cardiac failure or abdominal pain along with dyspnea, tachycardia, angina and unequal blood pressures on both sides. An aortic regurgitation murmur might be audible. CXR may reveal widened midiastinum. Echocardiogram, CT scan or MRI are used to diagnose dissection. It is a medical emergency and should be investigated and managed quickly to avoid mortality.

Types (Fig. 3.13)

- DeBakey:
    - Type I: Originating in ascending aorta but propagates beyond aortic arch.
    - Type II: Originating in ascending aorta but remains within aortic arch
    - Type III: Originating in descending aorta.

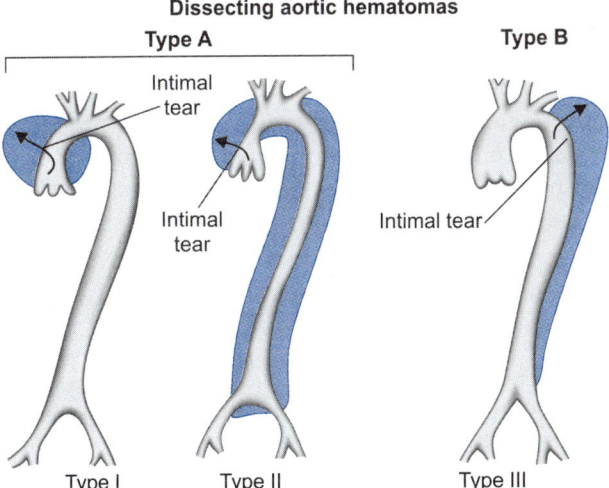

FIGURE 3.13: Dissecting aortic hematomas

- Stanford:
    - Type A: Involves ascending aorta and/or aortic arch. Includes DeBakey Type I and II
    - Type B: Involves descending aorta without involvement of the arch. Includes DeBakey Type III.

Aortic Dissection and Types

Causes

- Hypertension
- Hypercholesterolemia
- Coarctation of aorta
- Syphilis
- Trauma or instrumentation
- Marfan's syndrome or Ehler-Danlos syndrome.

Differential Diagnosis

- Myocardial infarction
- Pericarditis
- Pulmonary embolism
- Aneurysm.

Management

Close monitoring with control of blood pressure is extremely important. Initially, beta-blockers are preferred due to reduced inotropic effect and includes the use of esmolol and labetalol as infusions. Vasodilators can be added for resistant hypertension but can cause tachycardia. Calcium channel blockers like verapamil and diltiazem are used for the same reason. A mean arterial pressure of 60–75 mm Hg should be aimed for. Most dissections close to the heart will need surgery, while dissections away from the heart may be treated with blood pressure control alone. Endovascular devices are being used more and more now to avoid major surgeries. Immediate surgery is warranted in most cases of ascending aortic arch dissection; while others are treated conservatively unless organ damage is present. Pain relief is also important to reduce further damage and symptom relief.

Hypertensive Crisis

Diagnosis

Hypertensive crisis or emergency is hypertension with acute compromise of organ systems of the body like cardiovascular system, nervous system or renal system. Generally a blood pressure in the range of >240/130 mm Hg leads to signs and symptoms of end organ damage like angina, cardiac failure, hemorrhagic stroke, seizures, acute kidney injury amongst others warranting immediate treatment. This can also present as irritability, nausea, headache, confusion, chest pain and vision problems. On examination, apart from high blood pressure, tachycardia, retinal changes and neurological deficits might be present. Urine might show red cell casts or proteinuria; and ECG will show LVH with or without ischemic changes. In a young patient presenting like this, secondary causes of hypertension like pheochromocytoma, reno-vascular hypertension and drugs should be ruled out.

Management

In an hypertensive emergency with patients presenting with angina, myocardial infarct or stroke, blood pressure needs to be lowered quickly with drugs like labetolol, hydralazine or nitroprusside to prevent further damage. In other cases, the blood pressure is lowered gently over a few days to months. Drugs like ACE-inhibitors are useful in cardiac failure symptoms. If pheochromocytoma is suspected, use phentolamine before using beta-blockers. Nitroglycerin can also be used for heart failure and myocardial infarction. Investigations for end-organ damage should be carried out with CT, echocardiogram and ultrasound. This can then be followed up over time to check the response to medications.

Suggested Reading

1. Eraut D, Shaw DB. Sinus bradycardia. Br Heart J. 1971;33:742-9.
2. Gutierrez C, Blanchard DG. Atrial fibrillation: Diagnosis and Treatment. Am Fam Physician (Review). 2011;83(1):61-8.
3. Homback V, Hoher M, Kochs M, et al. Pathophysiology of unstable angina pectoris-correlations with coronary angioscopic imaging. European Heart Journal. 1988;9:40-5.
4. Isselbacher EM. Diseases of the aorta. In: Goldman L, Schafer AI, eds. Cecil Medicine. 24th Ed. Philadelphia, Pa:Saunders Elsevier; 2011:Chap 78.
5. John RM, Tedrow UB, Koplan BA. Ventricular arrhythmias and sudden cardiac death. Lancet. 2012;380(9852):1520-9.
6. LeWinter MM, Tischler MD. Pericardial disease. In: Bonow RO, Mann DL, Zipes DP, Libby P, eds. Braunwald's Heart Disease: A Textbook of Cardiovascular Medicine. 9th Ed. Philadelphia, Pa: Saunders Elsevier; 2011: Chap 75.
7. McMurray JJ, Pfeffer MA. Heart Failure. Lancet 2005; 365(9474):1877-89.
8. O'Gara PT, Kushner FG, Ascheim DD, et al. ACCF/AHA guideline for the management of ST-elevation myocardial infarction: a report of the American College of Cardiology Foundation/American Heart Association Task Force on Practice guidelines. Circulation. 2013;127:e362-e425.
9. Thomas L. Managing hypertensive emergencies in the ED. Can Fam Physician. 2011;57(10):1137-97.
10. Tobin KJ. Stable angina pectoris: What does the current clinical evidence tell us? J Am Osteopath Assoc. 2010;110(7):364-70.
11. Turi ZG. Mitral Valve disease. Circulation. 2004;109:e38-e41.
12. Wang PJ, Mark Estes III NA. Supraventricular tachycardia. Circulation. 2002;106:e206-e208.

CHAPTER 4

Renal Disorders in Intensive Care

Acute Kidney Injury

Acute kidney injury is a sudden reduction, but generally reversible decline in kidney function. This can result in an increase in creatinine, blood urea nitrogen (BUN) and other metabolic waste products. Two different systems of defining acute kidney injury exist: RIFLE (**r**isk, **i**njury, **f**ailure, **l**oss and **E**SRD) and AKIN (**a**cute **k**idney **i**njury **n**etwork) (Fig. 4.1).

Pathogenesis

Acute kidney injury can be due to pre-renal, renal and post-renal causes. Reduction in the urine output is common though not necessary. Most hospitalized patients will have acute tubular necrosis from sepsis, ischemia or toxins. Pre-renal cause due to dehydration or post-renal obstruction should always be ruled out as these are easily treatable causes leading to quick and complete recovery of renal function.

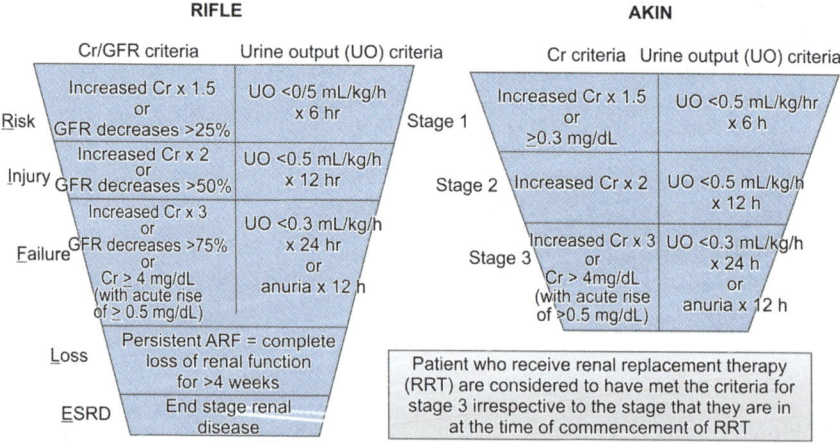

FIGURE 4.1: The AKIN and RIFLE definitions and grading for AKI

Diagnosis

Patients might present with lethargy, headache, confusion, encephalopathy and occasionally coma. In pre-renal azotemia, blood pressure may be labile with tachycardia and dry mucous membranes. Laboratory investigations may show academia and hyperkalemia. The blood urea nitrogen and creatinine will be raised. ECG may show arrhythmia and changes of hyperkalemia. Urine exam will show pus, crystals, Hb casts, bacteria, protein casts, etc. to distinguish between various causes.

Causes

Prerenal azotemia results from:
- Fluid depletion
- Diarrhea and vomiting
- Hypotension due to any cause
- Cardiac failure
- Drugs like diuretics, ACE-inhibitors.

Renal azotemia results from:
- Drug toxicity
- Acute tubular necrosis
- Glomerulonephritis
- Sepsis.

Post-renal azotemia results from:
- Obstruction caused by tumor
- Prostate enlargement
- Stones
- Clots
- Blocked urinary catheter.

Pre-renal and renal azotemia might be distinguished by fractional excretion of sodium: FeNa = [(urine Na × serum Cr)/(urine Cr × serum Na)] × 100. This will be <1% in pre-renal causes and >2% in ATN.

Complications

- Hyperkalemia
- Uremic encephalopathy
- Uremic pericarditis
- Fluid overload with oliguric renal failure
- Metabolic acidosis.

Management

- Fluid therapy should be considered in all cases. Crystalloids are preferred compared to colloids and should be used till physiological endpoints are reached.

- All nephrotoxic medications should be stopped like NSAIDs, aminoglycosides, ACE-inhibitors or ARBs.
- Dose adjustments for other drugs that accumulate in renal failure should be considered.
- Post-renal azotemia should be ruled out with ultrasound or CT scan as it is easily treatable and also gives an indication about the renal morphology.
- Renal biopsy is indicated in certain cases after specialist advice.
- In established renal failure unresponsive to fluids, renal replacement therapy should be considered.
  - The indications for dialysis/hemofiltration can be: hyperkalemia, hypovolemia, acidosis, encephalopathy, rapid rise in urea
- Acute acidosis and hyperkalemia can be treated while arrangements are made to start renal replacement therapy (RRT).

Golden Tips

- Fluids should be considered in all patients with acute kidney injury
- Ultrasound can be used to diagnose post-renal azotemia as it is surgically treatable
- Renal replacement therapy can be instituted for hyperkalemia, acidosis, hypovolemia and encephalopathy/pericarditis
- AKI is associated with increased morbidity and mortality in ICU patients and is an independent risk factor.

Renal Failure in Intensive Care Unit

Kidney injury in intensive care unit (ICU) is common and may be present in up to 50% of the patients. This is associated with increased healthcare costs and increased morbidity/mortality in the range of up to 50%.

Causes

There can be multiple causes of renal failure; some of which are preadmission while some occur in the ICU during the patients' stay. Preadmission volume depletion along with major surgery, sepsis, IV contrast, hepatic failure and various drugs are the common causes of renal failure in ICU patients. This leads to either pre-renal or renal azotemia.

Diagnosis

RIFLE and AKIN criterion are most commonly used to define the extent of renal injury. An ultrasound of the kidneys and urinary tract is advised in all the patients to rule out obstructive uropathy. Ultrasound can also give an idea of the renal size and possibility of chronic kidney problems too. If urinary catheter is in situ, accurate urinary output can be measured and kidney injury can be defined as oliguric or normo/polyuric renal injury.

Management

- Hydration should be checked and IV fluids administered in all cases unless there are contraindications
- Avoid all nephrotoxic medications like IV contrast, aminoglycosides, antifungals
- For any medication, check the appropriate dose based on the glomerular filtration rates
- If nephrotoxic medications have to be used, use formulations with lesser toxicity like liposomal amphotericin B or non-ionic contrasts
- Strict input output should be charted and fluid balance should be continuously monitored
- N-acetyl cysteine has shown some benefit with contrast induced nephropathy. Hydration remains paramount to avoid toxicity
- Albumin can reduce the incidence of renal injury in hepatic failure patients
- Managing the hemodynamics is more important than use of particular drugs like dopamine (renal dose)
- Diuretics should be used with caution (continuous infusion of furosemide may be better than bolus dose in patients with hemodynamic compromise).

Golden Tips

- Avoid further renal toxicity with drugs and medications
- Fluid balance should be managed strictly with set physiological goals
- Use less nephrotoxic formulations if possible
- Polyuric renal failure has lesser chance of needing renal replacement therapy.

Acute Tubular Necrosis

Acute tubular necrosis (ATN) is a type of acute kidney injury (AKI) where tubular network of kidneys is damaged. This is a very common cause of renal failure in ICU with high mortality. It can affect a large proportion of patients with sepsis, acute respiratory distress syndrome (ARDS) and multi-organ failure.

Causes and Symptoms

Acute tubular necrosis can result from hypoperfusion of the kidneys, hypotension, volume depletion, edematous states, drugs and IV contrast agents. Sepsis is a common culprit in many ICU patients. The symptoms are similar to acute kidney injury patients with malaise, oliguria/anuria, nausea, altered sensorium and coma. The kidneys lose ability to regulate electrolytes and water.

Diagnosis

It is sometimes difficult to differentiate pre-renal injury from acute tubular necrosis. This can be done by urinalysis, fractional excretion of sodium or response to fluids. The fractional excretion of sodium (FENa) is usually more than 2% and urine examination may show granular casts, some red or white cells. There is necrosis and denuding of epithelium into the tubules leading to casts and occlusion of the lumens. Other tests can be used for distinguishing these two like blood urea nitrogen (BUN)-creatinine ratio. Biomarkers are being developed for renal diseases too.

Management

- Prevention if possible will limit the morbidity and mortality of these patients
- Fluids can be tried to optimize and maximize the renal perfusion
- Avoid all nephrotoxic drugs and alter the dose of all drugs depending on the renal function and glomerular filtration rate
- Use of fluids and N-acetylcysteine before radiocontrast may reduce the number of patients needing renal replacement therapy
- Early recognition and institution of hemodialysis/hemofiltration can improve outcomes
- Close monitoring of electrolytes and volume status is essential. The initial oliguric phase may be followed by a polyuric phase where fluid balance has to be strictly monitored.

Golden Tips

- It can be difficult to distinguish between ATN and pre-renal AKI and they may coexist.
- Fluids should be still used as most patients will benefit from improved renal perfusion.
- FENA or other combination of tests can be used to distinguish between the two and direct treatment.

Rhabdomyolysis

Rhabdomyolysis is caused by muscle necrosis leading to release of intracellular contents into the circulation. This leads to myoglobinuria and renal damage along with muscular pain and a rise in creatine kinase (CK). Most patients recover completely from this as long as this is diagnosed and treated early.

Causes

- Traumatic muscular damage—crush or trauma
- Seizures
- Burns

- Malignant hyperpyrexia or neuroleptic malignant syndrome
- Tetanus
- Electrolyte imbalances like hypokalemia or hypophosphatemia
- Drugs like amphetamines, cocaine and statins
- Myositis
- Metabolic myopathies
- Severe exercise.

Pathophysiology

As the muscle cell dies, there is increase in intracellular calcium. This leads to rupture of membranes and extravasation of muscular proteins including myoglobin in blood. The myoglobin along with other muscle proteins are filtered through the glomerulus and cause tubular damage as they clump in the tubules leading to renal injury and acute tubular necrosis (ATN).

Diagnosis

Muscle tenderness may be present, but not necessary. Weakness is seen in some patients. There will be presence of dark urine in most patients. On urinanalysis there will be presence of heme without presence of red cells (heme and hemoglobin react with the strips). Laboratory findings include increased creatine kinase and other muscle enzymes like lactate dehydrogenase (LDH), aspartate aminotransferase (AST) and aldolase. The patients will present with rapid onset renal failure [rise in blood urea nitrogen (BUN) and creatinine] and its symptoms and symptoms from the cause like muscular pain, and weakness. Rule out presence of compartment syndrome and disseminated intravascular coagulation (seen in severe cases).

Management

- Fluid adequacy is important in the management of rhabdomyolysis. Fluid resuscitation remains paramount to reduce the damage to the tubules
- Once the fluid balance is restored, diuresis should be induced to flush out the myoglobin from tubules. This can be attempted with mannitol or furosemide
- Alkalinization of urine helps in dissolving the fragments and is achieved through use of sodium bicarbonate. A urine pH of >6.5 can be aimed for to reduce the cast formation. This can be difficult to achieve in some patients
- Renal replacement therapy may be needed in some patients where conservative management is not adequate.

Golden Tips

- CK is used to diagnose and guide management in rhabdomyolysis
- Fluid management is the most important intervention and urinary alkalinization can be tried to achieve a urinary pH >6.5
- Dialysis may be necessary in many cases.

Hepatorenal Syndrome

Hepatorenal syndrome refers to the acute kidney injury associated with acute or chronic liver disease patients. This represents the end-stage reduction in renal perfusion related to severe hepatic injury. This is ultimately a diagnosis of exclusion and can be associated with a high morbidity and mortality.

Diagnosis

This should be a diagnosis of exclusion after ruling out fluid depletion leading to prerenal failure, postrenal (obstruction) failure, or intrinsic renal failure [acute tubular necrosis (ATN), drugs, vasculitis]. On laboratory testing, high bilirubin, encephalopathy with signs of chronic hepatic failure like palmer erythema, varices and ascites in absence of shock, sepsis and nephrotoxic drugs and coagulopathy will be present. Renal failure exhibits as oliguria with fractional excretion of sodium (FENa) less than 1%.

Pathogenesis

Arteriolar vasodilatation in the splanchnic circulation triggered by portal hypertension plays a significant role in the pathophysiology. This in turn results into renal increase in renin or angiotensin system output and local vasoconstriction of renal vessels. Nitric oxide may be involved along with bacterial translocation in the initial response. The intense response of the kidneys leads to reduction in GFR and sodium absorption. This can be precipitated by bacterial infection, bleeds, or use of diuretics.

Types

- Type 1 shows a rapid rise in creatinine in a short period of time with reduced urine output and has poor prognosis
- Type 2 has resistant ascites but less severe disease.

Management

- Prevention remains important and albumin given in chronic hepatic failure may prevent development of hepatorenal syndrome
- All the nephrotoxic drugs should be avoided
- Intravascular volume should be restored if necessary with blood or albumin
- Sources of sepsis should be treated with appropriate antibiotics. Caution should be exercised as there is combined renal and hepatic failure in these patients
- Initial vasopressor treatment can be tried in very sick patients. Norepinephrine is the first agent of choice to target a specific blood pressure rise. Vasopressin can be used too
- If the patient is not very sick, terlipressin in bolus doses along with albumin can be tried

- Other agents like midodrine, octreotide and albumin are alternate agents
- Radiological interventions like transjugular intrahepatic portosystemic shunt (TIPPS) or LeVeen shunts have also shown anecdotal benefits
- Renal replacement therapy should be instituted in patients who are likely to survive or are waiting for transplantation
- Liver transplantation if appropriate will result in resolution of renal failure.

Golden Tips

- Hepatorenal syndrome is a diagnosis of exclusion carrying a high morbidity and mortality
- Treatment should aim at increasing the splanchnic vasoconstriction in turn improving the renal vasoconstriction
- Recovery of renal function is dependent on the recovery of hepatic function.

Pulmonary Renal Syndromes

Pulmonary renal syndromes are diseases that affect both the kidneys and the lungs. They generally consist of multisystem vasculitis with pulmonary and renal symptoms.

Presentation and Diagnosis

Patients may present with either pulmonary symptoms like cough, shortness of breath, hemoptysis; or with renal symptoms like renal failure, hematuria and loin pain. Many of these patients will also have other system disorders affecting skin, gastrointestinal or joints. Subsequent investigations will demonstrate pulmonary and renal affection. Chest X-ray (CXR) may demonstrate diffuse infiltrates or cavities, and broncho-alveolar lavage may show alveolar hemorrhage with macrophages. High resolution CT scan is useful in defining the lesions and helping in the diagnosis. Urine examination will demonstrate hematuria and casts. Blood markers like anti-neutrophil cytoplasmic antibodies (ANCA), antinuclear antibodies (ANA), ds-DNA, anti GBM may be positive depending on the etiology. Definitive diagnosis is usually by renal or lung biopsy.

Differential Diagnosis

Various diseases and syndromes leading to pulmonary-renal affection are:
- Wegener's granulomatosis
- Churg-Strauss disease
- Goodpasture's syndrome
- Microscopic polyangiitis
- Systemic lupus erythematosus
- Multisystem failure from other diseases like sepsis and congestive cardiac failure
- Drugs like amiodarone, procainamide, penicillamine, hydralazine, and quinidine.

Management

- Maintain airway, oxygenation and ventilation appropriately
- Many patients will need definitive airway due to the hemoptysis and pulmonary involvement
- Volume replacement and renal replacement therapy will also be needed in many cases
- Steroids have a role in most of these diseases
- Immunosuppression with azathioprine and cyclophosphamide is used in diseases like Wegener's granulomatosis
- Plasmapheresis is used in Goodpasture's syndrome with limited success.

Golden Tips

- Pulmonary renal syndromes are commonly caused by autoimmune disorders
- Glucocorticoids are the mainstay of treatment though immunosuppression is used in many of the diseases
- These diseases can have a very high early mortality, hence early diagnosis and treatment is essential.

Renal Replacement in Intensive Care Unit

Renal replacement therapy is used very commonly in the ICU. This can be used for both acute renal injury or chronic renal failure patients. The economic burden is high and use of renal replacement therapy has been linked independently to be a marker of increased mortality and morbidity.

Indications

- Acute renal injury
  - Hypervolemia leading to hemodynamic or respiratory compromise
  - Hyperkalemia sustained after conservative management
  - Acidosis
  - Uremic encephalopathy
  - Uremic pericarditis
  - Sustained rise in urea or creatinine
- Chronic renal failure
  - Associated with acute kidney injury with hemodynamic compromise
  - Chronic dialysis patients
- Poisoning or overdoses
  - Amitriptyline overdose
  - Methanol/alcohol overdose
- Other dialyzable molecules like myoglobin in rhabdomyolysis.

Types

Various forms of renal replacement can be used in ICU.

a. *Peritoneal dialysis*: This is the least commonly used method. Dialysis is done using peritoneum as the semipermeable membrane. Dialysate is introduced into the peritoneal cavity and after a set time, the fluid is removed (Fig. 4.2). It is unpredictable, slow and can lead to infection, bleeding, and injury to the gut. This can be used in patients already established on PD and are ready to be discharged to the ward/home as part of the rehabilitation.

b. *Hemodialysis*: A semi-permeable membrane is used and solutes move across by diffusion depending on the gradient (Fig. 4.3). This can be intermittent or continuous. Intermittent HD can lead to large fluid/electrolyte shifts and can be hemodynamically unstable. In ICU, continuous hemodialysis is used with lower flow rates to avoid this complication. It needs a secure intravenous access for the continuous flow of blood and the circuit needs to be anticoagulated because of this leading to the obvious complications like infection and bleeding. Heparin has been used for many years, though citrate has been shown to be better with lesser complications in recent trials.

c. *Hemofiltration*: In hemofiltration, the solutes and water move across by convection (*see* Fig. 4.3). The fluid lost is thus replaced back into the circuit.

Generally a combination of hemodialysis and hemofiltration are used in ICU settings. Both of these modalities need a central venous access and anticoagulation of the circuit. Modern machines can deliver both the modalities effectively in the ICU setting (Fig. 4.4)

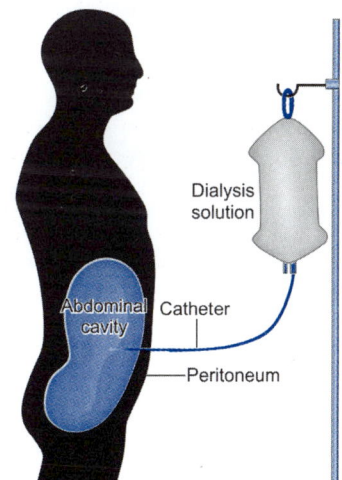

FIGURE 4.2: Set-up for peritoneal dialysis

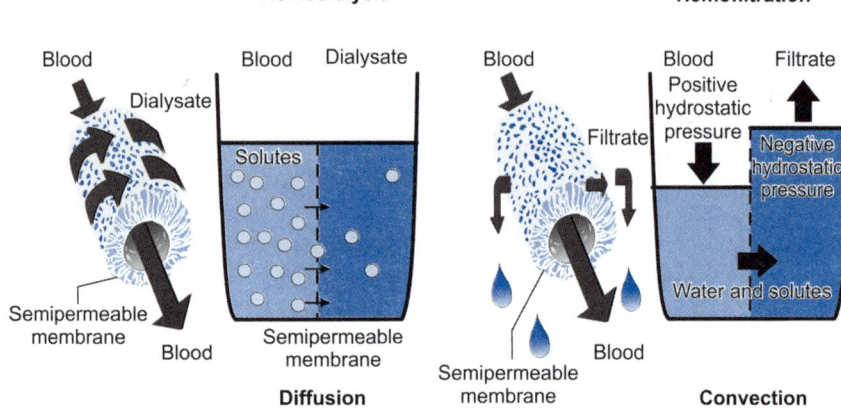

FIGURE 4.3: Renal replacement therapy

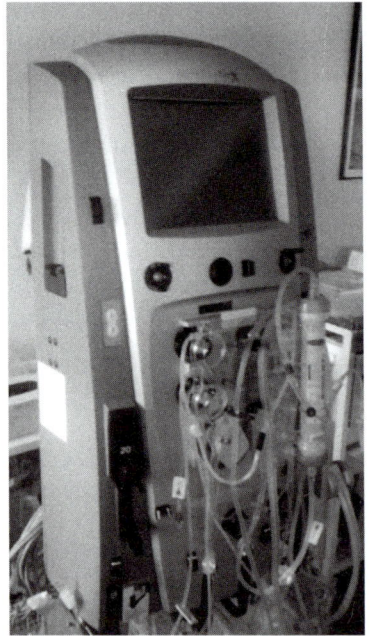

FIGURE 4.4: Modern hemodiafiltration machines for ICU use

Management

Central venous access as explained in Chapter 1. A double lumen wide bore access is needed for continuous flow at a high rate. Latest machines allow a lot of variables to be set including the flow rate, dialysate rate, anticoagulation rates, and net fluid balance to be maintained accurately. Continuous monitoring of hemodynamic variables is essential. Complications include infection, electrolyte and fluid imbalances, bleeding, hypotension and platelet consumption.

Golden Tips

- Renal replacement therapy is an essential part of ICU management
- Renal replacement therapy is an independent predictor of increased mortality and morbidity in ICU patients
- Various modalities can be used in patients depending on the clinical need and resources. Continuous and intermittent therapies have similar benefits.

Suggested Reading

1. Cruz DN, Ricci Z, Ronco C. Clinical review: RIFLE and AKIN- time for eappraisal. Crit Care. 2009;13(3):211-9.
2. Esson ML, Schrier RW. Diagnosis and treatment of acute tubular necrosis. Ann Intern Med. 2002;137:744-52.
3. Hoste EA, Schurgers M. Epidemiology of acute kidney injury: How big is the problem? Crit Care Med. 2008;36(4):S146-51.
4. KDIGO Clinicla Practice Guideline for Acute Kidney injury. Kidney Int Suppl. 2012;2(1):8-138.
5. Pannu N, Gibney RTN. Renal replacement therapy in the intensive care unit. Ther Clin Risk Manag. 2005;1(2):141-50.
6. Papiris SA, Manali ED, Kalomenidis L, et al. Bench-to-bedside review: Pulmonary-renal syndromes—an update for the intensivist. Crit Care. 2007;11:213-23.
7. Vanholder R, Sever MS, Erek E, Lameire N. Rhabdomyolysis. J Am Soc Nephrol. 2000;11:1553-61.
8. Wadei HM, Mai ML, Ahsan N, Gonwa TA. Hepatorenal syndrome: Pathophysiology and management. Clin J Am Soc Nephrol. 2006;1:1066-79.

CHAPTER 5

Essential Neurology

Guillain-Barre Syndrome

Guillain-Barre syndrome (GBS) is an immune mediated polyneuropathy generally provoked by a preceding infection. It is common in males compared to females and can vary in clinical progression and remission.

Infections Associated with Guillain-Barre Syndrome

- *Campylobacter jejuni*
- *Mycoplasma*
- *Cytomegalovirus*
- Varicella
- Hepatitis B.

Clinical Features

This is an acute ascending paralysis, which is flaccid in nature. It is predominantly motor affection, but paraesthesia and pain can be present with occasional cranial nerve or autonomic system affection. On examination, reflexes are diminished and pupils are spared. Around 10–30% will need some respiratory support. Pain is present in 2/3rd of patients and autonomic dysfunction in around 70%.

Diagnosis

- Cerebrospinal fluid (CSF) will reveal high proteins but normal white cell count (WCC) in about 2/3rd of patients
- Nerve conduction studies will demonstrate reduced velocity and axonal injury
- Antibodies like GQ1b, GM1, GD1a, GalNAc-GD1a and GD1b, GT1a, etc. are found in various forms of GBS.

Variants of Guillain-Barre Syndrome

- *Acute inflammatory demyelinating polyneuropathy*: It is the most common type with progressive symmetrical weakness with reduced reflexes

- *Acute motor axonal neuropathy*: This can be preceded by *Campylobacter jejuni* infection. Reflexes may be preserved and sensory system is not affected
- *Acute motor and sensory axonal neuropathy*: It is more severe than the above and has sensory involvement
- *Miller Fisher syndrome*: Ophthalmoplegia, ataxia and areflexia are present. Extension to extremity weakness may be present but is small. Antibodies to GQ1b are present.

Differential Diagnosis

- Myasthenia gravis
- Poliomyelitis
- Botulism
- Diphtheria
- Porphyria
- spinal cord transection
- Lambert-Eaton myasthenic syndrome
- Chronic inflammatory demyelinating polyneuropathy.

Management

- Respiratory capacity should be measured regularly as up to 30% patients need respiratory support. A vital capacity of <20 mL/kg, inspiratory pressure <30 cm H_2O or expiratory pressure <40 cm H_2O are indications for intubation
- Plasmapheresis or plasma exchange can remove circulating antibodies, complements and other agents leading to improvement in clinical condition
- Intravenous immunoglobulins have also been used and may modulate the antibody expression or produce an antagonistic affect leading to clinical improvement. It has been found to be more effective and safer than plasmaphersis
- Supportive care in the form of deep vein thrombosis (DVT) prophylaxis, nutrition, physiotherapy, gastric ulcer prophylaxis and general care are important as patients are limited in their mobility
- Autonomic dysfunction might need continuous monitoring as bradycardias and tachycardia can occur. Intravascular volume should be maintained. Beta-blockers or vasopressors are used to manage the swings in blood pressure and heart rates
- Pain should be adequately controlled. Tricyclic antidepressants, gabapentin or pregabalin have been used with success in these neuropathic pains.

Golden Tips

- Progressive weakness and areflexia are cardinal features of GBS
- Antibodies can be tested to distinguish between different variants of GBS

- Plasma exchange or intravenous immunoglobulin (IVIG) can be used with success in severe GBS
- Steroids should not be used in the treatment of GBS.

Myasthenia Gravis

Myasthenia gravis is a neuromuscular disorder resulting from development of antibodies to the acetylcholine receptors. It has a bimodal distribution with young females and old males affected more commonly.

Pathophysiology

Development of antibodies results in attack to the postsynaptic membrane of neuromuscular junction. Any stress or infection can precipitate the crisis. Many patients have associated thymoma. Myasthenia can be generalized and ocular.

Clinical Features

- Fluctuating weakness
- Only skeletal muscles affected
- No sensory symptoms and reflexes are normal
- Fatigue and increased symptoms with day progression
- Eyes are commonly affected with diplopia/ptosis common.

Diagnosis

- Edrophonium test reveals improved motor function and nerve conduction will demonstrate decreased response with repeated stimulus
- Acetylcholine receptor (AChR) antibodies will be present in 90% of generalized myasthenics and 50% of ocular myasthenics. Muscle specific tyrosine kinase (MuSK) antibodies are also present in up to 50% patients. This can be associated with other auto-immune diseases like thyrotoxicosis, polymyositis, rheumatoid disease and systemic lupus erythematosus (SLE)
- CT scans of the chest is done in patients to rule out presence of thymoma.

Differential Diagnosis

- Guillain-Barre syndrome (GBS)
- Botulism
- Lambert-Eaton myasthenic syndrome
- Myopathies
- Motor neuron disease.

Management

- Monitoring of vital capacity is again essential. Ventilatory support may be needed if it drops below 20 mL/kg. Supportive measures as in GBS should be used in acute situations.

Essential Neurology

- Anticholinesterase inhibitors are the mainstay of symptomatic treatment. Pyridostigmine is used for benefit of long half-life and oral formulation. This increases the availability of acetylcholine to the receptors.
- Corticosteroids and immunosuppressants are used for immunomodulation.
- For acute state, plasma exchange or intravenous immunoglobulin can be used.
- Thymectomy in the presence of thymoma can offer long-term benefits. Timing of surgery should be based upon clinical situation and IVIG or plasma exchange can be tried before surgery to optimise the patient.

Golden Tips

- Myasthenia is an autoimmune disorder that may be associated with other autoimmune disorders
- Treatment consists of symptom relief, chronic immunomodulation, acute treatment with plasmapheresis or intravenous immunoglobuline (IVIG) and consideration of thymectomy
- Myasthenic and cholinergic crisis can occur and can be difficult to differentiate. Edrophonium can be used to distinguish between the two.

Muscular Dystrophy

Muscular dystrophies are a group of disorders leading to progressive myopathies due to genetic defects. The primary symptom is muscle weakness. The most common diseases are Duchenne and Becker muscular dystrophy.

Diagnosis and Presentation

This presents as progressive muscular wasting and weakness. It is more pronounced in the proximal muscles and occasionally presents with hypertrophy of the muscles. There is an increased use of hands to support for standing from a sitting position refered to as 'Gower's sign'. This can be associated with cardiac conduction anomalies and cardiomyopathy, and mental impairment. Duchenne dystrophy presents early, while the symptoms for Becker dystrophy present later and are milder. In limb-girdle dystrophy, the pseudo-hypertrophy of muscles is not seen that often. Laboratory findings will include elevated creatine kinase. This will eventually settle over years as muscle is replaced by fibrous tissue. Aldolase levels will be raised too. Muscle biopsy will show necrosis, macrophage infiltration and fat deposits in the muscles. ECG will show tall R waves in right leads with increased R/S ratio and deep Q waves in I, aVL and V5-6 leads. There may be presence of conduction abnormalities and increased QRS duration. EMG will show myopathic changes (polyphasic potentials).

Genetics

These diseases are caused by defective dystrophin gene on the X-chromosome leading to defect in the dystrophin protein. In Duchenne disease, the reading frame is disrupted, while in Beckers disease the coding sequence is maintained.

Differential Diagnosis

- Myasthenia gravis
- Guillain-Barre syndrome (GBS)
- Motor neuron disease
- Polymyositis
- Pyomyositis
- Botulism
- Poliomyelitis.

Management

This is a progressive disorder with no treatment:
- Glucocorticoids remain the mainstay of treatment and are recommended in all boys 5 years and older. This reduces the progression, but may delay puberty and stunt growth. Prednisone is beneficial in improving the functionality
- Deflazacort is a derivative of prednisolone and has been shown to be equally efficacious with possible better side effect profile
- Respiratory insufficiency should be treated with early non-invasive ventilation and invasive ventilation considered as per the wish of the patient. Tracheostomy is considered early for long-term support
- Cardiac complications may need cardiology opinion with regards to placement of permanent pacemaker or defibrillator for conduction abnormalities
- Careful consideration to the type of anesthetic is essential as these patients may react abnormally to some drugs
- Consideration should be given to nutrition as drugs can cause weight gain and osteopenia leading to fractures.

Golden Tips

- Mutation in dystrophin gene on X-chromosome leads to Duchenne and Becker muscular dystrophy
- Elevated creatine kinase (CK), electrocardiogram (ECG) changes and muscle biopsy is generally sufficient to characterize the disease
- Steroids are the mainstay of treatment currently, though new therapies including gene therapy, cell therapy and new drugs are undergoing trials.

Critical Illness Polyneuropathy

Critical illness polyneurophathy is characterized by neuromuscular weakness in critically ill patients and can affect 1 in 4 patients especially if they were ventilated for >7 days. This can occur due to the severe disease, but also because of drugs like steroids and muscle relaxants.

Diagnosis

Commonly seen in patients with prolonged intensive care unit (ICU) stay, more commonly in severe sepsis with multiorgan failure and acute respiratory distress syndrome (ARDS). The suspected mechanism is decreased microcirculation of distal nerves leading to axonal degeneration. This presents with sensori-motor polyneuropathy with sensory deficits with pinprick and touch, weakness and atrophy, loss of reflexes pointing towards peripheral neuropathy. The cranial nerves are preserved. Nerve conduction study (NCS) shows features of generalized axonal sensorimotor polyneuropathy with reduced action potentials, loss of motor units, demyelination and conduction blocks. Direct muscle stimulation will show increased amplitude. Serum creatine kinase (CK) is normal and muscle biopsy will show neurogenic dystrophy.

Differential Diagnosis

- Rhabdomyolysis
- Medications like amphotericin, muscle relaxants, neuroleptics, etc.
- Cachexia
- Guillain-Barre syndrome (GBS)
- Botulism
- Critical illness myopathy.

Management

- Supportive treatment is needed in severe cases and this may take months to years to resolve or may not resolve completely
- Intensive insulin therapy has been shown to lower incidence of polyneuropathy
- Cause should be treated aggressively to prevent prolonged ventilation and multiorgan failure
- Nutrition, electrolyte imbalances and avoidance of neurotoxic drugs are important during rehabilitation.

Golden Tips

- One in four patients with severe sepsis may experience critical illness polyneuropathy which may take months to years to resolve

- Intensive blood glucose control may be linked with reduced incidence of critical illness polyneuropathy, but may be in turn increase mortality
- Can be differentiated from myopathy by muscle biopsy and direct muscle stimulation along with nerve conduction studies.

Critical Illness Myopathy

Critical illness myopathy is a form of myopathy seen in critical illness patients that is commonly found in about 1/3rd patients admitted with respiratory disease like chronic obstructive pulmonary disease (COPD) or acute severe asthma. It is also seen in patients with liver transplant, and may be related to systemic use of corticosteroids in these patients. A smaller group of patients have had paralytic agent exposure; while high blood sugars, hyperthyroidism and SIRS may contribute too.

Diagnosis and Presentation

This presents as flaccid paralysis of proximal muscles and failure of ventilator wean. Sensations are generally normal and reflexes are normal too. This can occur in conjunction with polyneuropathy. Muscle biopsy is diagnostic and creatine kinase (CK) may be elevated. Nerve conduction studies are essentially normal, though neuropathy can coexist. Primary muscular disorders, nutritional deficiencies, drugs like statins, electrolyte abnormalities and thyroid disorders should be ruled out.

Management

- Correction of underlying disorder should be the primary aim
- Avoidance of systemic steroids can prevent the complication
- Electrolyte correction, nutrition, physiotherapy should be done in all cases
- Glucose control can lower the incidence of myopathy, but has the risk of increasing mortality in the critical care setting.

Golden Tips

- Critical illness myopathy is most strongly linked with use of systemic steroids
- This can be reversible but may take months to years for that and increase intensive care unit (ICU) and hospital stay
- Intensive glucose treatment may reduce the incidence of myopathy.

Head Injury

Head injury or traumatic brain injury is one of the leading causes of death in young population. The survivors are left with significant disability. This can also be associated with other injuries that may need more urgent attention.

Diagnosis and Presentation

The mechanism of injury along with the location and extent are paramount for management of head injury cases. The presentation may be from asymptomatic to coma; most patients present with skin laceration/wound, headache, nausea/vomiting, amnesia or loss of consciousness. Examination may be normal or there might be pupillary signs, bruising (Battle sign or raccoon eyes), focal neurology, decreased Glasgow Coma Scale (GCS) or coma. Injuries are related to the mechanism and force of injury and include skull fracture, concussion, cerebral contusion, axonal injury, and traumatic hemorrhage. This can then lead to raised intracranial pressure, secondary ischemia, electrolyte imbalance, hypoxia and hypotension. GCS should be done frequently and pupils checked regularly. Computed tomography (CT) scan is diagnostic, but some cases might require MRI. Spinal injuries are associated in many cases.

Glasgow Coma Scale

Eye opening	Points
Eyes open spontaneously	4
Eyes open to verbal command	3
Eyes open only with painful stimull	2
No eye opening	1

Verbal response	
Oriented and converses	5
Disorented and converses	4
Inappropriate words	3
Incomprehensible sounds	2
No verbal response	1

Motor response	
Obeys verbal commands	6
Response to painful stimull (UE)	
Localize pain	5
Withdraws from pain	4
Flexor posturing	3
Extensor posturing	2
No motor response	1

Total score = eye opening + verbal + motor
   GCS <5: 80% die or remain vegitative
   GCS >11: 90% complete recovery

Source: Teasdale G, Jennett B. Acta Neurochirurg. 1976;34:45.

Management

Prehospital care: Hypoxia should be prevented and blood pressure maintained. Early endotracheal intubation should be considered if resources available when GCS is <8. Supplemental oxygen and IV fluids in the form of crystalloids should be used preferably.

Emergency department: A systematic approach should be considered in all cases of head injury. Airway should be secured with control of cervical spine in suspected cases if already not done. If the GCS is <8 or there is associated airway trauma, early intubation is indicated. Oxygenation is important in all cases of head trauma. Control of ventilation and $paCO_2$ at a low normal levels is ideal if increased intracranial pressure is suspected. Mean arterial pressure should be maintained as normal as possible and IV fluids should be started. Attention should be paid to other associated injuries and advanced trauma life support (ATLS) algorithms can be very useful in such situations. Imaging in the form of X-rays, CT scans and ultrasound should all be done in a focused manner in the emergency department. Lab tests should be ordered including complete blood count (CBC), electrolytes, coagulation studies and blood should be sent for typing and crossmatch.

ICU management: Oxygenation and blood pressure maintenance remains important. IV fluids are given as appropriate and albumin should be avoided in traumatic brain injury. Intracranial pressures (ICP) can be measured either directly or indirectly based on the available resources. External ventricular drain, subdural or extradural bolts and ultrasound have all been used for this. Depending on the clinical condition and direct measurements, the treatment is instituted:

- *Maintaining blood pressure*: Blood pressure should be maintained for cerebral perfusion. Systolic blood pressure >90 mm Hg should be maintained. Crystalloids should be used for resuscitation
- *Oxygenation*: Maintain PaO_2 >60 mm Hg. Oxygenation is important to reduce the delayed ischemic injury
- Raised ICP:
  - Head of bed should be elevated to 30 degrees
  - Keep neck in neutral position
  - Improve venous drainage by removing constrictive dressings/tapes
  - Osmotic therapy with mannitol and hypertonic saline can be used in acute situation. Monitor the osmolality (keep <320 mMol/L) and Na levels (keep <155)
  - Hyperventilation to a $PaCO_2$ of 30 mm Hg has been used as a temporizing measure. Hypocarbia can lead to vasoconstriction and can be detrimental in some patients
  - Sedation and paralysis: These have been used in cases of uncontrolled increase in ICP. Pharmacological agents vary from propofol and benzodiazepines to barbiturates
  - Hypothermia: Hypothermia down to a temperature of 32 degrees has been used in refractory cases
  - Surgery: Surgical intervention is needed for hematoma evacuation, removal of foreign bodies, fractures and ventricular drain placement. Decompressive craniectomy can be done in selected patients.

- Maintain glucose control as both increased and decreased blood sugars are associated with worse outcomes
- Steroids should be avoided in traumatic brain injury
- Antiepileptics can be used for early seizures for 7 days.

Golden Tips

- GCS <8 is considered as severe traumatic brain injury and will need airway control
- Surgical intervention is based on clinical finding and extent of injury
- ICP should be targeted below 20 cm H_2O.

Intracranial Hypertension

The normal pressure in the intracranial compartment is <15 mm Hg. A rise in this pressure to >20 mm Hg is considered as pathological.

Causes

- Traumatic brain injury
- Space occupying tumor
- Hydrocephalus
- Stroke
- Subarachnoid hemorrhage
- Hepatic encephalopathy.

Monro-Kellie Doctrine

The intracranial space is a rigid bony space with a fixed volume of 1400–1700 cc. It contains three things:
- Brain: 80%
- Blood: 10%
- CSF: 10%

The presence of any other pathology like abscess, tumor or hematoma will change this equilibrium leading to either displacement of one of the above components or an increase in intracranial pressure. As brain parenchyma will have a fixed volume, the major changes occur in blood and CSF. The rise in volume is compensated by decrease in blood and CSF volume to a certain extent (critical volume) after which even small rise in pathological volume will lead to steep rise in intracranial pressure (Fig. 5.1).

Cerebral Perfusion Pressure

This is the clinical measure for adequate perfusion in the brain.
$$CPP = MAP-ICP$$
where, Cerebral perfusion pressure (CPP); mean arterial pressure (MAP); intracranial pressure (ICP).

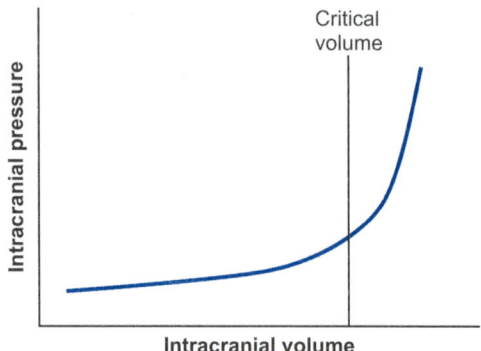

FIGURE 5.1: Graph of intracranial pressure to volume (note the sudden rise in pressure after reaching critical volume)

Cerebral blood flow (and perfusion) is auto-regulated over a wide range of CPP (50–100 mm Hg). This is altered in pathologies like trauma and stroke.

Diagnosis and Presentation

Common presentations are:
- Headache
- Nausea or vomiting
- Reduced GCS
- Pupils may be abnormal with VI nerve affected commonly leading to mydriasis
- Abnormal posturing and respiratory response
- Abnormal neurological findings
- Cushing's triad is a late finding (hypertension, bradycardia and abnormal breathing pattern)
- CT and MRI might show space-occupying lesion in the brain with midline shift, edema, decreased ventricular size, effacement of sulci amongst others; but direct ICP measurement is diagnostic (this has been discussed in another chapter).

Management

- Urgent evaluation of the possible cause and resuscitation with fluids and oxygen should be done
- Airway control is important in comatose patients. A secure airway will help with control of $paCO_2$ to control ICP.
- Large swings in blood pressure should be managed with fluids and vasopressors to achieve a MAP of >90 mm Hg
- Patient's head should be elevated
- Mannitol, furosemide and hypertonic saline can all be used to control the ICP in acute situations; along with hyperventilation to a $paCO_2$ below

normal range. Once this is stabilized, hyperventilation should be tapered towards normalcy
- Sedation can reduce the oxygen demand and reduce ICP
- Corticosteroids useful only in malignancy, some CNS infections or post-operatively in some cases. They may be harmful in other cases
- Hypothermia and barbiturate coma with burst suppression can be tried if the above fails for short period
- CSF drainage procedures like ventricular drain are used in cases where its feasible
- Surgery (decompressive craniectomy) is limited to patients where medical management fails.

Golden Tips

- ICP is regulated as per the Monro-Kellie doctrine and can rise sharply with small changes in volume after critical volume is reached
- Temporary measures like osmotics, hyperventilation, hypothermia and deep sedation are used to decrease the ICP
- Steroids offer no benefit in trauma or stroke, but may be helpful in tumors, some infections and postoperatively.

Stroke

Stroke is a general term used for any cerebrovascular accident. This leads to sudden loss of brain function in most patient.

Types of Stroke (Fig. 5.2)

- Hemorrhagic stroke
- Ischemic or thromoembolic stroke
- Subarachnoid hemorrhage.

Presentation

The symptoms depend on the area of the brain or territory affected. Hemorrhagic strokes are sudden and usually associated with nausea/vomiting and headache. Most patients will have a history of hypertension. It is also common in patients on warfarin or other anticoagulant drugs. The most common sites for hemorrhagic stroke are basal ganglia, cerebellum, thalamus and pons. Any other site should raise suspicion about a different etiology like aneurysm, AV malformation, tumor or amyloid disease.

Embolic strokes have maximum deficit at the beginning of the symptomatic period and then might improve over time as the embolus is dislodged or lysed. Thrombotic strokes on the other hand are sudden and may evolve over time. The presentation can vary from minor motor or sensory deficit to aphasia, hemiparesis/hemiplegia, impaired speech or cerebellar dysfunction.

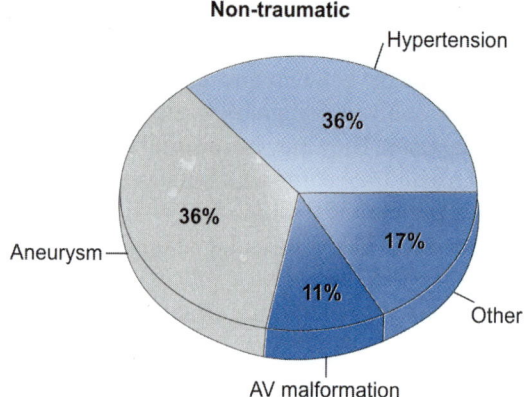

FIGURE 5.2: Major causes of intracerebral hemorrhage

Other causes: Bleeding into tumor, hypocoagulable state, hemorrhagic infarction, iatrogenic, and trauma

Diagnosis

CT scan or MRI are mandatory in any stroke. CT is very sensitive for hemorrhagic stroke, but not for acute ischemic stroke. MRI is sensitive for ischemic and posterior fossa lesions. This should be differentiated from hypoglycemia, tumors, seizure, migraine and vasculitis.

Other tests such as blood glucose, ECG, cardiac enzymes, serum chemistry panel and coagulation studies should be done for further management. Oxygen saturation should be monitored in all patients.

The risk factors for all strokes are hypertension, diabetes, smoking, arteriopathy, ischemic cardiac disease and arrhythmias.

Management

- Airway and breathing should be assessed and managed first.
- Fluids should be started as many patients will be fluid deplete. Free water in the form of dextrose should be avoided.
- Blood sugars should be maintained in normal range. Both hypoglycemia and hyperglycemia should be treated
- Treat any coagulation or platelet abnormality that might have led to stroke
- Blood pressure should be maintained and hypertension should not be treated aggressively. A sudden reduction in blood pressure in the first 24 hours may be detrimental.
- If thrombolytic therapy is being planned in ischemic stroke, a blood pressure of <185/110 mm Hg should be maintained and maintained below 180/105 mm Hg for another 24 hours. If this is not planned the blood

pressure should be maintained below 220/120 mm Hg unless there is another reason to control it.
- Neurology should be assessed regularly. For hemorrhagic stroke, physiological parameters should be maintained.
- Surgical advice can be sought for posterior fossa bleeds and may be helpful occasionally for other major bleeds.
- Ischemic strokes should be given aspirin and tissue plasminogen activator or alteplase should be considered as per local protocols. Intra-arterial thrombolysis can be considered in selected patients. Again, physiological variables should be maintained as normal as possible.
- Antithrombotic therapy and DVT prophylaxis should be considered for ischemic strokes.
- Statins and blood pressure control is considered along with advise on lifestyle, smoking, diabetes and hypertension.
- Signs of intracranial hypertension should be treated as previously described.

Golden Tips

- Imaging should be done immediately to define type of stroke
- Fluid and glucose management should be started and patients scanned for thrombolytic therapy
- Blood pressure should not be lowered rapidly.

Subarachnoid Hemorrhage

About 10% of the strokes are due to subarachnoid hemorrhage (SAH). Most of these are caused by ruptured saccular aneurysms in the cerebral circulation. These can have significant mortality and morbidity associated with SAH, but with better care this is improving.

Diagnosis

Patients describe a sudden severe headache—'worst headaches of their life'; occasionally preceded by warning headache few hours to days before the actual event. This is associated with nausea, vomiting, neck stiffness, pain and loss of consciousness on occasions. On examination, neck stiffness may be present along with signs of intracranial hypertension, symptoms of stroke depending on the site of SAH. 'Terson's syndrome' is presence of preretinal hemorrhage and indicates poor prognosis. CT scan is the first line diagnostic tool and may show the bleed; occasionally lumbar puncture may be required. Blood or xanthochromia will be present. Cerebral angiogram may be required for the site and presence of vasospasm. Digital substraction angiography or CT/MR angiography are used to define the lesion.

Grades of Subarachnoid Hemorrhage (Tables 5.1 and 5.2)

Table 5.1: Hunt and Hess classification of SAH

Grade	Criteria	Index of perioperative mortality (%)
0	Aneurysm is not ruptured	0–5
I	Asymptomatic or with minimal headache and slight nuchal rigidity	0–5
II	Moderate of severe headache, nuchal rigidity, but no neurologic deficit other than cranial nerve palsy	2–10
III	Somnolence, confusion, medium focal deficits	10–15
IV	Stupor, hemiparesis medium or severe, possible early decerebrate rigidity, vegetative disturbances	60–70
V	Deep coma, decerebrate rigidity, moribund appearance	70–100

Table 5.2: World Federation of Neurosurgeon's grading

WFNS grades	GCS score	Motor deficit
I	15	Absent
II	14–13	Absent
III	14–13	Present
IV	12–7	Present or absent
V	6–3	Present or absent

Interpretation

- Maximum score of 15 has the best prognosis
- Minimum score of 3 has the worst prognosis
- Scores of 8 or above have a good chance for recovery
- Scores of 3–5 are potentially fatal, especially if accompanied by fixed pupils or absent oculovestibular responses.

Complications

- Rebleeding: 5–25% patients rebleed mostly within 24 hours
- Vasospasm and ischemia: can occur in up to 50% patients
- Hydrocephalus: 10–15% of the patients
- Intracranial hypertension
- Seizures.

Differential Diagnosis

- Stroke
- Meningoencephalitis
- Migraine.

Management

- Airway and breathing should be assessed and controlled. Intubation may be required in appropriate cases. The indications include GCS <8, poor pulmonary function, hemodynamic instability and increased ICP
- Hemodynamics should be stabilized with tight blood pressure control. IV fluids should be started to prevent hypovolemia
- Deep vein thrombosis (DVT) prophylaxis should be started and heparin/low-molecular-weight heparin (LMWH) is added after securing the aneurysm
- Bed rest, pain relief and quiet settings will be needed
- Hyperglycemia, fevers, anemia, myocardial ischemia and other fluid and electrolyte abnormalities should be treated appropriately
- Blood pressure is preferably managed <160 mm Hg before securing aneurysm and anti-epileptics are used in patients who have seizures
- Depending on the neurological examination, early surgical intervention may be required in the form of clipping or coiling. Coiling is tried in easy to reach aneurysms with small necks; others require craniotomy and clipping.
- In presence of vasospasm, nimodipine (60 mg four times a day) is used and euvolemia is maintained. Triple H therapy (hypervolemia, hemodilution and hypertension) may be used in selected symptomatic cases of vasospasm with use of vasopressors. Statins have also been used in such cases.
- Hydrocephalus may need placement of ventricular drain
- Supportive management in the form of nutrition, electrolyte management and ulcer prophylaxis.

Golden Tips

- About 10% of the strokes are due to SAH
- There is a high chance of rebleeding in the first 24 hours and vasospasm for many days
- Nimodipine has been shown to improve morbidity and mortality and triple H therapy can be tried in selected patients
- First degree relatives of SAH patients have an increased chances of SAH and can be screened for presence of aneurysms.

Altered Sensorium

This remains a common problem in all ICU patients, especially elderly patients. It can be hard to recognize and has significant morbidity and mortality associated with this.

Definition

Delirium is defined as:
- Disturbed consciousness with decreased ability to focus, sustain or shift attention

- Changed cognition or perceptual disturbance not related to dementia
- Fluctuating and short duration of disturbance
- Evidence of relation to medical condition, intoxication or drugs
- Psychomotor disturbances with hypo or hyperactivity, sympathetic disturbances and sleep disturbances
- Varied emotional changes.

Risk Factors

- Dementia
- Stroke
- Parkinsonism
- Advanced age and sensory impairment
- Drugs like anticholinergics, dopamine agonists, anticonvulsants, opioids, antidepressants, etc.
- Infection/sepsis
- Dehydration
- Malnutrition.

Presentation

Nearly 30% of older medical patients will develop delirium during hospitalization. ICU patients have a much higher rate. The patients can be hyperactive or hypoactive. There is disturbance in conscious level and drowsiness, change in perception and memory loss of orientation are common findings. Associated signs may be present in the form of hypertension, tachycardia, tachypnea, dyssynchronous breathing and difficulty in weaning. These signs appear relatively quickly over hours to days compared to months to years in dementia. It is also common in elderly and demented patients and can confuse the diagnosis.

Diagnosis

If the patients are partially sedated, this may be very difficult to evaluate and recognize. Methods used to assess this are mini mental state examination, confusion assessment method for intensive care units (CAM-ICU) (Fig. 5.3). Intensive Care Delirium Screening Checklist (ICDSC) can also be used and correlates well with CAM-ICU. Medical conditions leading to delirium should be investigated and treated appropriately. All sources of infections should be ruled out and fluid electrolyte and metabolic parameters normalized.

Management

- All medical causes of delirium should be investigated and treated before treatment of altered sensorium is considered.
- If the patient is a danger to others or himself, treatment for delirium should be started.

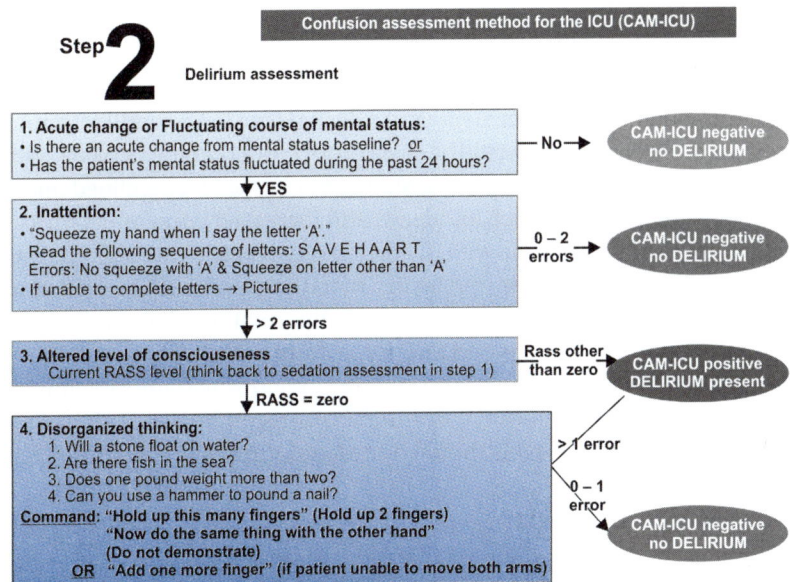

FIGURE 5.3: CAM-ICU scoring sheet

- Drugs like haloperidol and clonidine have been tried with success.
- Family and relatives should be asked to stay around as much as possible to reduce confusion and orientate the patient.
- Benzodiazepines can also be tried for withdrawal or seizures, but have limited role in delirium otherwise.
- Other antipsychotics like olanzapine, quetiapine, risperidone and ziprasidone have also been tried.

Golden Tips

- Delirium is a complex condition related to medical diagnosis, substance intoxication or drug effect with reduced consciousness and lack of attention
- Up to 70% of ICU patients may suffer from delirium during their stay
- All physiological parameters should be normalized and treatment can be started in severe cases
- There is no role of prophylactic medication in delirium.

Coma

Coma is a state of decreased responsiveness to external stimuli to the point of being unarousable. Stupor is decreased responsiveness where the patient is still arousable.

Diagnosis

Glasgow Coma Score (GCS) is used commonly in all patients with impaired responsiveness. A GCS of less than 8 can be used as definition of coma. This can be due to various lesions in the brain or a generalized depressed function of the brain due to systemic causes affecting the ascending reticular activating system. The patients may present with papillary dysfunction, abnormalities in eye movements, motor abnormalities like flexion or extension and respiratory asynchrony. Neck stiffness should be checked to rule out central nervous system (CNS) infections or bleed and fundus should be checked for papilloedema. CT scan will be required to check for bleeds and increased intracranial pressure (ICP). Bloods should be done with full metabolic screen to rule out electrolyte abnormalities, renal function and toxins. Blood sugars should be carried out. Occasionally MRI is required for structural abnormalities. Lumbar puncture is used to diagnose infections and EEG for seizures, which may be subclinical. Adrenal and thyroid function tests, cultures, blood smear for disseminated intravascular coagulation (DIC) or thrombotic thrombocytopenic purpura (TTP) and specific drug levels should be ordered if the cause remains elusive.

Differential Diagnosis

- *Psychogenic*: with resistance to eye opening, atypical seizures, distinguished eye movements
- *Locked-in syndrome*: with preserved consciousness but loss of motor function with injury to pons. Eye movements are preserved
- *Akinetic mutism*: prefrontal or premotor cortex areas lead to loss of ability to move, but they follow with the eyes. Reflexes are preserved.

Management

- Airway and breathing should be assessed and managed first. Most comatose patients will need airway protection in the form of endotracheal tube if the GCS is <9, unless the diagnosis is clear and treatment rapid
- Hypotension should be treated with fluids and vasopressors as required
- Dextrose and thiamine can be given while waiting for further blood tests
- Intracranial hypertension is managed as described before
- Most patients will need a CT scan and a lumbar puncture once other common causes are ruled out
- Naloxone and flumazenil are tried if opioid or benzodiazepine overdose is suspected
- Antibiotics and antivirals are used in suspected meningitis
- Antiepileptics are given if seizures are suspected while this is investigated.

Golden Tips

- There are multiple causes of coma due to various disease processes
- Prompt airway control is important to preserve brain function-in acute situations glucose with thiamine can be given and naloxone/flumazenil considered depending on the presentation.

Status Epilepticus

Status epilepticus is single continuous seizure lasting 5-10 minute or frequent seizures without normalization of mental state in between seizures. This can be refractory to treatment with initial medications and leads to increased morbidity.

Types of seizures are:
- Primary generalized seizures
    - Absence seizures: Abrupt with body tone maintenance, eye movements and spontaneous complete recovery
    - Myoclonic seizures: Presence of myoclonic jerks
    - Atonic seizures: Loss of tone and abrupt fall
    - Tonic seizures: Hypertonia
    - Clonic seizures: Presence of clonus
    - Tonic-clonic seizures: Combination of above
- Partial seizures
    - Simple partial: No loss of consciousness
    - Complex partial: Loss of consciousness
    - Secondary generalized seizure.

Precipitating factors like non-compliance with drugs, ischemia, infections, withdrawal, drugs, hypoxia, metabolic disorders and tumors should be ruled out. CT scan and lumbar puncture hence may be required in first time presenters. EEG is diagnostic during an acute episode.

Management

- Identify the precipitating causes as above and treat
- Acute control is with benzodiazepines. Diazepam is a stable drug and has fast onset of action, but lasts for a shorter time due to redistribution. Lorazepam is slow in onset but lasts longer. Midazolam can be used as an infusion for refractory epilepsy
- Phenytoin can also be used as first line treatment and has the added advantage of suppressing seizures for longer time. Fosphenytoin has better solubility and side effect profile
- Valproic acid, levetiracetam, topiramate, lacosamide and fosamax are being used more often now because of better side effect profile
- Airway and breathing should be evaluated and controlled in prolonged seizures
- In status uncontrolled with benzodiazepines and phenytoin, consider intubating and sedating with propofol. EEG monitoring should be used and if still in status, barbiturates or benzodiazepine infusion can be considered and expert opinion sought.

Golden Tips

❑ Status epilepticus can have multiple etiologies including noncompliance, previous structural defects, trauma, stroke and infections
❑ Lorazepam is the recommended first line agent, while phenytoin and valproic acid along with newer agents being used more often now.

Suggested Reading

1. Bederson JB, Connolly ES Jr, Batjer HH, et al. Guidelines for the management of aneurysmal subarachnoid hemorrhage: a statement for healthcare professionals from a special writing group of the Stroke Council, American Heart Association. Stroke. 2009;40:994-1025.
2. Broderick J, Connolly S, Feldmann E, et al. Guidelines for the management of spontaneous intracerebral hemorrhage in adults: 2007 update—from the American Heart Association/American Stroke Association, Stroke council, High blood pressure Research council and the Quality of Care and Outcomes in Research Interdisciplinary Working Group. Stroke. 2007;38:2001-23.
3. Bullock MR, Povlishock JT (Ed). Guidelines for the management of severe traumatic brain injury. J Neurotrauma. 2007;24(suppl 1):S1-S106.
4. Emery AE. The muscular dystrophies. Lancet. 2002;359(9307):687-95.
5. Gerace RV, McCauley WA, Wijdicks EF. Emergency management of the comatose patient. In: Coma and Impaired Consciousness: A Clinical Perspective. Young GB, Ropper AH, Bolton CF (Eds). McGraw Hill, New York .1998;P 563.
6. Jauch EC, Savel JL, Adams HP Jr, et al. Guidelines for the early management of patients with acute ischemic stroke: a guideline for healthcare professionals from the American Heart Association/American Stroke Association. Stroke. 2013;44:870-947.
7. Lassen NA, Christensen MS. Physiology of cerebral blood flow. Br J Anaesth. 1976;48:719-34.
8. Latronico N, Bolton CF. Critical illness polyneuropathy and myopathy: a major cause of muscle weakness and paralysis. Lancet Neurol. 2011;10(10):931-41.
9. Meierkord H, Boon P, Engelsen B, et al. EFNS guideline on the management of status epilepticus. Euro Jour Neurol. 2006;13(5): 445-50.
10. Skeie GO, Apostolski S, Evoli A, et al. Guidelines for treatment of autoimmune neuromuscular transmission disorders. Eur J Neurol. 2010;17(7):893-902.
11. Van den Boogaard M, Schoonhoven L, Evers AW, et al. Delirium in critically ill patients: impact on long-term health-related quality of life and cognitive functioning. Crit Care Med. 2012;40(1):112-8.
12. Yuki N, Hartung HP. Gullian-Barre syndrome. N Engl J Med. 2012;366(24):2294-304.

CHAPTER 6

Fluid and Electrolyte Disorders

Hypernatremia

Hypernatremia is a common problem in intensive care unit (ICU) patients. This generally results from deficiency of water in relation to the sodium. If the ingested water lags behind this loss, hypernatremia can result. Some of this may be iatrogenic due to wrong choice of fluids or therapeautic [as in treatment for raised intracranial pressure (ICP)].

Signs and Symptoms

The patient may complain of lethargy, weakness or irritability, but with more severe rise seizures and coma may result. The severe symptoms occur at levels >155 mEq/L, while the normal levels are between 135–145 mEq/L. A serum sodium of more than 145 mmol/L defines hypernatremia.

Causes

- Hypovolemia
    - Reduced free water intake in elderly or disabled
    - Excess loss in urine as in diabetes (with sodium loss) or diuretics
    - Extreme heat and sweating
    - Severe diarrhea
- Euvolemia
    - Diabetes insipidus leading to water loss
- Hypervolemia
    - Hypertonic saline or sodium bicarbonate infusion
    - Conn's syndrome
    - Excessive salt intake.

Management

- Avoid further hypertonic solutions and treat the underlying cause of hypernatremia
- Estimate the total water deficit and correct the Na slowly. It is recommended to correct this slowly at the rate of 10 mmol/day as rapid correction may lead to cerebral edema with subsequent risk of seizures, brain damage and death

- Water deficit = total body water × difference in Na/normal Na
- If hypovolemic, correct with isotonic solutions
- Hypernatremia in presence of fluid overload like congestive cardiac failure or renal failure may require hemodialysis for Na correction.

Hyponatremia

Diagnosis

Hyponatremia is present when the serum Na is less than 135 mEq/L. Severe hyponatremia is defined as levels below a level of 125 mEq/L symptoms can range from nausea, vomiting, headache, confusion, lethargy, fatigue, irritability, stupor and coma. Seizures may be present and depend on the rapidity of change in the concentration. Again assessing the volume status and checking the serum and urine osmolality is important for treatment.

Types

- Hypervolemic hyponatremia
  - Cirrhosis
  - Nephrotic syndrome
  - Congestive cardiac failure
  - Primary polydipsia
- Euvolemic hyponatremia
  - Syndrome of inappropriate antidiuretic hormone secretion (SIADH)
  - Hypothyroidism
  - Steroid deficiency
  - Trauma and brain injury
- Hypovolemic hyponatremia
  - Prolonged vomiting, diarrhea or reduced intake
  - Addison's disease
  - Diuretics.

Management

- Correction of hyponatremia will depend on the chronicity of the problem
- If the hyponatremia is recent, rapid correction can be achieved; but in chronic states, correction should be 8–10 mEq/L/day
- In a hypovolemic patient, the extracellular volume replacement should be achieved. Otherwise fluids should be restricted to 1–1.5 L/day and this will lead to slow correction of hyponatremia
- For SIADH, demeclocyline can be considered
- Underlying cause should be treated
- If the sodium is corrected rapidly, there are chances of developing central pontine myelinolysis with high-risk in alcoholics and malnourished patients

Fluid and Electrolyte Disorders

- Vasopressin receptor antagonist (vaptans) can be used in patients with SIADH, congestive cardiac failure or liver cirrhosis.

Hyperkalemia

Diagnosis and Causes

Elevation of potassium in the blood is called hyperkalemia. K levels are maintained within a range of 3.5–5 mEq/L in the blood. Hence a level of >5 mEq/L is hyperkalemia. Severe hyperkalemia is a medical emergency and can lead to fatal cardiac arrest. At lower levels, nonspecific symptoms like malaise, palpitations, muscle weakness is present. ECG may show tall T waves, reduced P amplitude, prolonged PR, wide QRS, sine waves and eventually ventricular fibrillation (Fig. 6.1).

Causes

- Reduced elimination
  - Renal impairment
  - Adrenal insufficiency
  - Medications like ACE-inhibitors, diuretics (spirononlactone), NSAIDs, trimethoprim, etc.
  - Gordon's syndrome
  - Renal tubular acidosis.
- Increased release from cells
  - Blood transfusion or hemolysis
  - Acidosis leading to K shifts
  - Rhabdomyolysis
  - Use of succinylcholine
  - Tumor lysis
  - Burns.
- Increased intake
  - Dietary supplements
  - Iatrogenic.

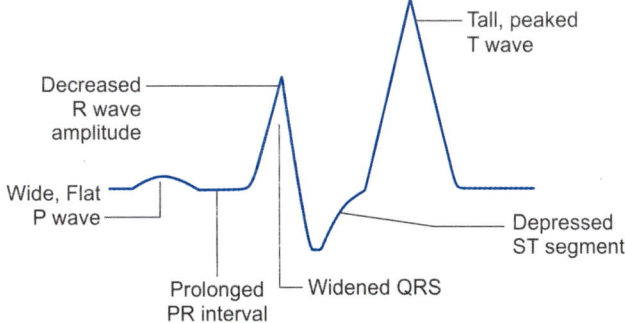

FIGURE 6.1: ECG changes in hyperkalemia

Management

- If acute ECG changes present, calcium gluconate or chloride give cardiac protection
- Sodium bicarbonate can be tried to shift potassium intracellularly
- Nebulized salbutamol can be helpful for short-term as this shifts the K intracellularly too
- Insulin with dextrose also has the same effect and it lasts for a few hours while the cause is treated
- Loop diuretics and oral potassium binding resins can decrease the potassium
- Hemodialysis is a very efficient method of controlling the potassium and is needed in many patients
- Potassium should be limited in the diet and medications.

Hypokalemia

Serum potassium <3.5 mEq/L is defined as hypokalemia. This can be asymptomatic, but muscle weakness, dyspnea, paralytic-ileus, hypotension can all be present. Rhabdomyolysis can occur at levels <2 mEQ/L. ECG may show flat T waves, presence of U waves, ST depression, AF, ventricular arrhythmia, tachycardia and fibrillation (Fig. 6.2).

Causes

- Inadequate intake
    - Starvation
    - Low potassium diet
- Increased extra-renal loss
    - Diarrhea
    - Perspiration
    - Vomiting

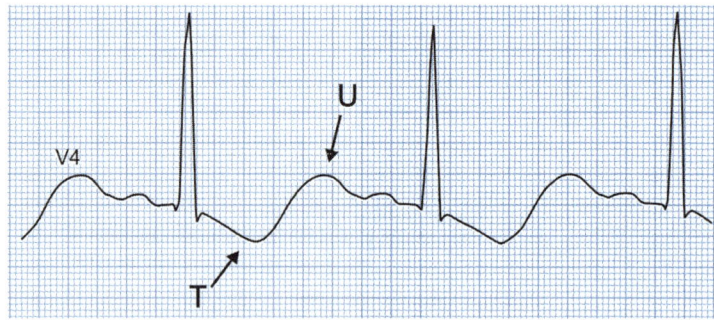

FIGURE 6.2: ECG changes in hypokalemia

- Increased renal loss
  - Diuretics, antifungals
  - Diabetes ketoacidosis
  - Hypomagnesemia
  - Alkalosis (intracellular shift and renal loss)
  - High aldosterone levels
  - Bartter's and Gitelman's syndrome
- Others
  - Alkalosis
  - Hereditary defects
  - Medications like salbutamol and insulin.

Management

- Find and treat the cause of hypokalemia
- Replacement can be oral or intravenous
- Mild hypokalemia can be treated with oral supplementation and fruits and vegetables should be advised to the patients
- Severe hypokalemia requires intravenous supplementation. This can be done at fast rates only through central venous access
- Potassium sparing diuretics like amiloride or spironolactone can be used in resistant cases
- With the presence of renal impairment, caution should be exercised due to chances of accumulation.

Hypercalcemia

Calcium levels in blood are maintained between 9–10.5 mg/dL. Hypercalcemia is a calcium level above 10.5 mg/dL. It can be asymptomatic or can be associated with anorexia, nausea, vomiting, ileus, constipation, abdominal pain, pancreatitis, altered sensorium, psychosis and coma. Renal effects include polyuria, polydipsia and stones. There is increased fracture risk and ECG will demonstrate short QT interval and occasionally arrhythmias in digitalized patients (Fig. 6.3).

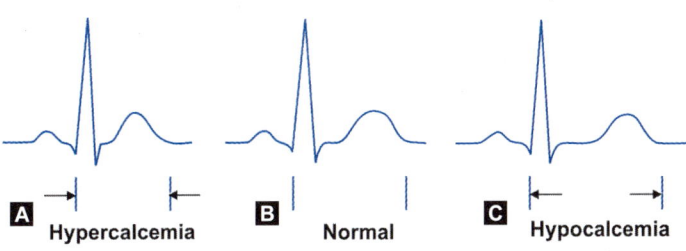

FIGURE 6.3: ECG changes in hypercalcemia and hypocalcemia

Causes

- Abnormal parathyroid function
    - Primary hyperparathyroidism
    - Secondary and tertiary hyperparathyroidism
- Malignancy
- Vitamin D disorders
- Renal impairment
- Milk alkali syndrome
- Hyperthyroidism
- Drugs like thiazide diuretics
- Multiple myeloma
- Immobilization
- Calcium supplements
- Sarcoidosis.

Management

- Assess and treat the cause of hypercalcemia
- Fluid resuscitation will lead to volume expansion and loss of calcium through the kidneys
- Loop diuretics can be tried after volume expansion
- In life threatening or symptomatic hypercalcemia, calcitonin can be given but the effects are short lived
- Bisphosphonates can lower the calcium slowly over days
- Steroids can be used in sarcoidosis or malignancy
- Hemodialysis is the most effective way to lower calcium in many cases.

Hypocalcemia

Hypocalcemia is presence of low calcium in the blood. Calcium levels <8.5 mg/dL can lead to symptoms and signs of hypocalcemia. This can present as tetany, increased reflexes, paresthesia, weakness, altered sensorium and seizures. Increased reflexes may be seen as Chvostek's sign (tapping on facial nerve leads to grimacing) and Trousseau's sign (blood pressure measurement leads to carpopedal spasm). ECG may show prolonged QT interval and cardiac contractility may be reduced and arrhythmias precipitated.

Causes

- Hypoparathyroidism
- Renal impairment
- Pancreatitis
- Sepsis
- Vitamin D and calcium deficiency

- Tumor lysis syndrome
- Rhabdomyolysis
- Diuretic therapy
- Massive transfusion
- Hypomagnesemia, hyperphosphatemia
- Alkalosis due to hyperventilation
- Post-parathyroidectomy surgery.

Management

- Find and treat the underlying cause
- Intravenous calcium can be given in acute situations
- Oral calcium can be used for slow replacement along with vitamin D
- If renal losses are high, consider thiazide diuretics
- Magnesium should be corrected if associated deficiency
- Consider hungry-bone syndrome if phosphates are low after parathyroidectomy; while hypoparathyroidism if elevated.

Hypermagnesemia

Serum magnesium levels more than 3.7 mg/dL is considered high. This may lead to diminished reflexes, muscle weakness, respiratory failure, vasodilatation and hypotension. It progresses to reduced consciousness and coma at high levels. ECG will show prolonged QT, conduction defects, heart blocks and asystole.

Based on serum concentrations various signs and symptoms may result:
- 4 mEq/L: hyporeflexia
- >5 mEq/L: prolonged AV conduction
- >10 mEq/L: complete heart block
- >13 mEq/L: cardiac arrest.

Causes

- Renal failure
- Increased intake (laxatives and antacids)
- Hemolysis
- Diabetes, adrenal insufficiency, hyperparathyroidism, lithium intoxication
- Treatment of eclampsia disorders and tetanus
- Hypothyroidism
- Addison's disease
- Milk alkali syndrome.

Management

- Identification and treatment of the cause is important
- Avoid all fluids containing magnesium

- Acute cardiac effects can be reversed by calcium gluconate or chloride
- Hemodialysis is rarely needed in extreme situations
- Regular deep tendon reflexes should be examined when administering magnesium.

Hypomagnesemia

A serum magnesium level less than 0.7 mg/dL signifies hypomagnesemia. It presents with weakness, cramps, tremors, tetany, and altered mentation at severe deficiency. Various cardiac arrhythmias may be precipitated including ventricular tachycardia and torsades de pointes.

Causes

- Dietary deficiency as in alcoholics and chronic diarrhea
- Medications like diuretics, antibiotics (aminoglycosides), proton-pump inhibitors, digoxin, etc.
- GI tract losses in Crohn's disease, ulcerative colitis and Whipple's disease
- Vitamin D deficiency
- Renal tubular acidosis/Fanconi's syndrome
- Refeeding syndrome
- Malabsorption
- Diabetes
- Association with other electrolyte abnormalities like hypocalcemia, hypokalemia and metabolic alkalosis
- Thyrotoxicosis.

Management

- As magnesium is primarily intracellular, the replacement needed may be huge
- Underlying cause should be treated and magnesium replaced slowly in renal failure
- Oral replacement can be used in mild deficiency, but many ICU patients will need intravenous replacement. It has also become essential treatment in various cardiac arrhythmias, asthma and preeclampsia in the ICU. If other electrolytes are low, magnesium should be corrected simultaneously for better effect.

Hyperphosphatemia

Diagnosis and Causes

Serum phosphate >5 mg/dL can cause symptoms of hyperphosphatemia. It is generally asymptomatic, but along with hypocalcemia can cause tetany, seizures, hypotension and arrhythmias. The calcium salt may get deposited in various organs leading to conduction system defects, renal stones and lung problems.

It is generally caused by:
- Impaired renal excretion due to renal failure, parathyroid disorders, heparin therapy or acromegaly
- Increased extracellular phosphate load as in exogenous administration, crush injury, tumor lysis, rhabdomyolysis, increased intake or ingestion in drugs and enemas.

Management

- Identify and treat the cause
- Avoid further phosphate administration in any form
- If asymptomatic, there is no need to treat
- In symptomatic patients, volume should be restored and diuretics can be tried
- In chronic cases, phosphate binders can be tried
- Hemodialysis can be considered in selected cases
- If the product of calcium and phosphate is more than 70, risk of calcification is high.

Hypophosphatemia

Diagnosis and Causes

Serum phosphate of <2.5 mg/dL is diagnostic of hypophosphatemia although most cases will be asymptomatic at this level. Muscle weakness, respiratory failure, impaired hematopoietic function, rhabdomyolysis, altered mentation, stupor and coma, seizures, etc. can all occur; more so at levels < 1.5 mg/dL. This is more common in alcoholics, severe malnutrition, refeeding syndrome, diabetes with insulin dependence, hyperparathyroidism, hypercalcemia, reduced vitamin D, antacids, phosphate binders, renal transplant, and Fanconi's syndrome. Any alkalemic condition (specifically respiratory alkalosis) will also reduce phosphate from the plasma. Malabsorption and antacid use can also lead to phosphate deficiency.

Management

- The cause of hypophosphatemia should be identified and treated promptly
- Oral phosphate replacements are used in patients with no or mild symptoms
- Intravenous phosphates are used in severe cases. This should be done slowly over few hours to reduce chances of calcification
- Other electrolyte abnormalities should be treated appropriately.

Hypervolemia

Diagnosis

Hypervolemia is presence of increased fluid- this may be generalized or localized. This may present as peripheral edema, ascites, pulmonary edema with or without pleural effusions, shortness of breath, hypoxia, cyanosis or altered mentation. This can be associated with decreased, increased or normal intravascular volume. Hypervolemia is seen in congestive cardiac failure, nephritic syndrome, cirrhosis, hypoalbuminemia due to any cause, sepsis, increased sodium intake, and can be iatrogenic.

Management

Underlying cause should be identified and treated. Diuretics can be tried if renal function is stable. Sodium and fluids should be restricted as appropriate. Ascitis if present can be drained and replaced with albumin to reduce reaccumulation. For respiratory problems, supplemental oxygen should be given and diuretics tried. Pleural effusion drainage is of limited benefit unless the cause is corrected. In cardiogenic edema, preload and afterload should be reduced to decrease the myocardial oxygen demand. Morphine, diuretics, ACE-inhibitors, nitroglycerine, sodium nitroprusside may be needed. Noninvasive ventilation or CPAP may be of benefit in the short-term; failing which invasive mechanical ventilation may be required. Hemodialysis is considered in resistant cases.

Hypovolemia

Diagnosis and Causes

This is defined as reduced effective circulating volume. This can present as thirst, dry mucous membranes to confusion, lethargy and coma. Postural drop in blood pressure may be the first sign of dehydration. This can lead to shock and multiorgan failure if not treated. The central venous pressure will be low and renal function will be altered. This can result from excessive loss as in vomiting, diarrhea, sweating; increased renal loss in diabetes mellitus and insipidus, diuretic use, polyuric renal failure, burns, internal or external hemorrhage, reduced intake in psychiatric problems, dementia or reduced consciousness, adrenal insufficiency or hepatic, cardiac or renal failures.

Management

Identification of the cause is important in deciding the type of fluid to be used for resuscitation. This can be a crystalloid, colloid or blood products. The resuscitation can be guided by patient symptoms or use of various parameters like heart rate, blood pressure, central venous pressure or other cardiac output monitors. Regular review of hemodynamic state and the fluids infused should be done to avoid overload and electrolytes should be measured regularly.

Suggested Reading

1. Adrogue HJ, Madias NE. Hypernatremia. N Engl J med. 2000;342(20):1493-9.
2. Assadi F. Hypophosphatemia: an evidence-based problem-solving approach to clinical cases. Iran J Kidney Dis. 2010;4(3):195-201.
3. Diercks DB, Shumaik GM, Harrigan RA. Electrocardiographic manifestations: electrolyte abnormalities. J Emerg Med. 2004;27:153-60.
4. Makras P, Papapoulos SE. Medical treatment of hypercalcaemia. Hormones. 2009;8(2):83-95.
5. Martin KJ, Gonzalez EA, Slatopolsky E. Clinical consequences and management of hypomagnesemia. J Am Soc Nephrol. 2009;20(11):2291-5.
6. Musso CG. Magnesium metabolism in health and disease. Int Urol Nephrol. 2009;41(2):357-62.
7. Prie D, Beck L, Urena P, Friedlander G. Recent findings in phosphate homeostasis. Curr Opin Nephrol Hypertens. 2005;14:318-24.
8. Sarko J. Bone and mineral metabolism. Emerg Med Clin North Am. 2005;23(3):703-21.
9. West ML, Marsden PA, Richardson RM, et al. New clinical approach to evaluate disorders of potassium excretion. Miner Electrolyte Metab. 1986;12(4):234-8.
10. Zenenberg RD, Carluccio AL, Merlin MA. Hyponatremia: evaluation and management. Hosp Pract. 2010;38(1):89-96.

CHAPTER 7

Acid and Base Disorders

Metabolic Acidosis

Acid-base balance is strictly controlled by the presence of buffers in the body, renal and respiratory systems. The quantity of acid in the body is measured in pH which is $= -\log[H^+]$. Arterial pH is constantly maintained between 7.35–7.45.

Definition

A pH <7.35 with decrease in the bicarbonate ions in blood due to increased H^+ ions is referred as metabolic acidosis. The presence of metabolic acidosis can be due to increased acid production, loss of bicarbonate ions or decrease in acid excretion by the kidneys.

Causes for Metabolic Acidosis

- Increased generation of acid
    - Ketoacidosis with diabetes mellitus, alcohol or malnutrition
    - Ingestion of methanol, ethylene glycol, aspirin, etc.
    - Lactic acidosis.
- Loss of bicarbonate
    - Diarrhea
    - Ureteral diversion procedures
    - Type 2 RTA.
- Decreased excretion
    - Renal impairment
    - Type 1 RTA.

There may be a decrease in $paCO_2$ as the respiratory system tries to compensate. The symptoms are tachypnea, fatigue, weakness, lethargy, sleepiness, coma and abdominal pain. This in severe cases can lead to shock, vasoplegia, cardiac failure when the pH <7.15. Potassium leaks out of the cells and leads to hyperkalemia.

Diagnosis

Serum and urine anion gap can be calculated to diagnose the cause (Na- HCO_3^- Cl). Normal serum gap is 12 ± 4 for serum and 0 for urine. If urine anion gap is >0, the cause for the acidosis is likely renal cause. High anion gap acidosis can be due to high lactic acid, renal failure, ketoacidosis, toxins like aspirin overdose, and rhabdomyolysis; while non-anion gap acidosis is due to renal tubular acidosis, hypoaldosteronism, and diarrhea.

Management

- Identify and treat the underlying cause
- Correct the fluid and electrolyte imbalances
- Severe symptomatic acidemia can be corrected with sodium bicarbonate infusion to keep the pH >7.2 as pH below this can lead to resistant hypotension and other adverse consequences
- Chronic acidosis can be treated with alkali therapy once the cause is known
- For continued metabolic acidosis, hemodialysis is the stabilizing measure while the primary problem is corrected.

Golden Tips

- Metabolic acidosis can result from increased production, decreased elimination or loss of bicarbonate from the body
- Serum anion gap can be used to distinguish it into high anion gap and normal anion gap acidosis
- Treatment with bicarbonate can be initiated as stabilizing measure while the cause is treated.

Metabolic Alkalosis

Diagnosis and Presentation

Metabolic alkalosis is a rise in pH due to metabolic conditions either because of a decrease in hydrogen ions leading to increased proportion of bicarbonate ions or a direct rise in bicarbonate ions. Thus it exists with an increase in serum bicarbonate and an arterial pH >7.45. The clinical features are paresthesia, tetany, lethargy, confusion, seizures and occasional hypoventilation with increased $paCO_2$. Tachycardia and hypotension can be present along with arrhythmias. Hypertension can be seen in specific conditions like glucocorticoid usage or Cushing's syndrome.

Causes

- Chloride responsive (urine chloride <20 mEq/L):
  - H^+ loss due to vomiting (may be associated with hypokalemia or hyponatremia)
  - Chloride diarrhea
  - Contraction alkalosis (diuretic usage)
  - Hypercapnia when corrected may lead to metabolic alkalosis
  - Cystic fibrosis.

- Chloride resistant (urine chloride >20 mEq/L):
  - Bicarbonate retention
  - Hypokalemia (cellular shift of H⁺ ions for electrical neutrality)
  - Iatrogenic with IV fluids, antacids
  - Hyperaldosteronism (Conn's syndrome)
  - Cushing's syndrome
  - Bartter, Gitelman, Liddle syndromes
  - Toxicity with antibiotics like aminoglycosides.

Management

Once the cause is identified, treatment can be instituted appropriately. In chloride responsive cases, normal saline should be used to restore volume. In chloride resistant states, cause should be identified. In mineralocorticoid excess disorders, spironolactone may be used. Electrolytes should be corrected and acetazolamide may be used with caution after volume loading in selected cases.

Golden Tips

- Alkalosis results from either removal of H⁺ ions or excess of HCO_3^- ions in the blood
- Contraction alkalosis occurs with the use of diuretics losing bicarbonate-free fluid and hence a relative excess of bicarbonate in the blood.

Respiratory Acidosis

Diagnosis and Causes

Respiratory acidosis results from decreased ventilation leading to an arterial pH <7.35 with elevated $paCO_2$. If this is chronic, there will be a compensatory rise in the bicarbonate ions by the kidneys. Respiratory acidosis may lead to somnolence, headache, tremors, confusion, coma, incordination, respiratory fatigue and failure.

Causes

- Acute:
  - Stroke/coma
  - Trauma to spine or chest
  - Neuromuscular diseases like myasthenia gravis, Guillain-Barre syndrome (GBS), motor neuron disease (MND)
  - Iatrogenic with inadequate ventilator settings
  - Drugs like sedative drugs, opioids, alcohol
  - Airway obstruction
  - Muscle relaxants or inadequate reversal

- Electrolyte imbalances
- Organophosphorus poisoning.
- Chronic:
  - Chronic obstructive pulmonary disease (COPD)
  - Obesity hypoventilation syndrome
  - Chronic inflammatory demyelinating polyneuropathy (CIDP), myasthenia gravis
  - Pulmonary fibrosis
  - Thoracic deformities.

Compensation

The renal system compensates for the change in CO_2 because of the acidosis. The average compensation in acute respiratory acidosis is 1 mEq/L for every 10 mm Hg increase in $PaCO_2$, while in chronic acidosis it is 3.5 mEq/L for every 10 mm Hg increase.

Management

The main treatment is to identify and treat the cause for acidosis. Avoid drugs that can worsen respiration. Many patients will need non-invasive or invasive mechanical ventilation. Normalization of pH should be the initial aim of treatment, while $PaCO_2$ will take longer to normalize. Permissive hypercapnia may be needed in many such cases.

Golden Tips

- Respiratory acidosis can result from a number of diseases affecting the nervous system, muscles or lung parenchyma.
- The renal system takes longer to compensate for the acidosis and this may not be complete for a few weeks.
- Identification and treatment of the cause is important.

Respiratory Alkalosis

Diagnosis and Causes

Increased ventilation leading to a decrease in H^+ (via removal of CO_2) is referred to as respiratory alkalosis if the arterial pH >7.45. This can lead to a secondary compensation through the renal system whereby the HCO_3^- ions are excreted in the urine. This can present as confusion, irritability, paraesthesia, seizures and coma. Arrhythmias can be present with other nonspecific ECG changes.

Causes

- Central hyperventilation syndrome
- Hypoxia

- Pulmonary fibrosis
- Pulmonary edema
- Anxiety
- Pain and fever
- Salicylate toxicity
- Pregnancy (physiological)
- Iatrogenic hyperventilation
- High altitude
- Stroke.

Compensation

- In acute respiratory alkalosis, HCO_3^- ions drop by 2 mEq/L for every 10 mm Hg drop in $PaCO_2$
- In chronic respiratory alkalosis, HCO_3^- ions drop by 5 mEq/L for every 10 mm Hg drop in $PaCO_2$.

Management

Identification of the cause is again important. Once the cause is treated, the acid base disturbance corrects. If the patient is intubated and ventilated, arterial blood gases (ABGs) should be used to guide the ventilator settings. In severe symptomatic cases, control of ventilation may be required to avoid drastic acid base disorder.

Mixed Acid–Base Disturbances

Diagnosis

This is a coexistence of two or more disorders together. This can present as normal pH with abnormal $paCO_2$ and HCO_3^-. pH will change in opposite direction of the primary disorder. Anion gap >20 mmol/L indicated primary metabolic acidosis. Determine corrected bicarbonate and pH. Any deviation from 7.4 will tell us what the primary disorder is. Respiratory compensation is checked to confirm the combination of disorders. This can be respiratory and metabolic acidosis as in cardiac arrest or respiratory with renal failure; respiratory and metabolic alkalosis as in pregnancy with hyperemesis, over ventilation in chronic obstructive pulmonary disease (COPD); respiratory alkalosis with metabolic acidosis as in sepsis, salicylate poisoning, etc.

Management

Identify the primary and secondary causes as above and treat the cause.

Suggested Reading

1. Murray J, Nadel J. Hypoventilation syndromes. In: Textbook of Respiratory Medicine. 4th Ed. Philadelphia, Pa. WB Saunders. 2005;(2):2075-80.
2. Palmer BF. Metabolic alkalosis. Jour Amer Soc Nephrol. 1997;8(9):1462-9.
3. Rose BD, Post TW. Clinical physiology of acid-base and electrolyte disorders. 5th Ed, McGraw-Hill, New York. 2001;583.

CHAPTER 8

Shock

Sepsis and Septic Shock

Septic shock is a systemic response to severe infection. This can lead to multiple organ dysfunction and death. The mortality rate from septic shock remains high even with all the advances in treatment.

Definition

- Systemic inflammatory response syndrome (SIRS):
  - At least 2 of the following:
    - Tachypnea >20/minute or $PaCO_2$ <32 mm Hg on arterial blood gas (ABG)
    - White cell count (WCC) <4000 or >12000
    - Heart rate > 90 beats/minute
    - Temperature >38 or <36.
- Sepsis:
  - SIRS resulting from suspected or proven infectious source like positive blood culture, CXR or other findings.
- Severe sepsis:
  - Signs of end-organ dysfunction like renal injury, liver dysfunction, mental changes, rise in lactate, coagulation abnormalities, etc.
- Septic shock:
  - Refractory hypotension even after adequate fluid resuscitation.

Presentation

The patients will present with hypotension and hypoperfusion to the end organs. Apart from the above systemic features, organ damage presents with altered mental status, respiratory and cardiovascular instability, liver derangements, acute kidney injury and deranged coagulation. The lactate levels will rise due to tissue perfusion problems and is used in the goal directed therapy. Initial warm peripheries due to vasodilatation. This will initially present with reduced peripheral resistance, increased cardiac index, tachycardia and hypotension; but may be affected later with cardiac failure.

Differential Diagnosis

❏ Other types of shock like hypovolemic, cardiogenic, obstructive and anaphylactic shock.

Management

Once severe sepsis or septic shock are recognized, time is of essence. The management should begin in accordance with the surviving sepsis guidance. Rapid assessment and initiation of treatment is essential. Blood cultures should be taken along with cultures from suspected sources and broadspectrum antibiotics started based on local guidance and suspected organisms. Fluids should be administered to correct for hypovolemia. Urine output should be measured regularly and response to fluids gauged. Lactate levels can be used for goal directed therapy. Central venous pressure monitoring may be required for fluid requirement and institution of vasoactive therapy. If hypotension persists, noradrenaline is the drugs of choice. If respiratory failure ensues, ventilatory support may be required. Vasopressin may be required in resistant cases and renal replacement therapy for renal impairment and acidosis.

Surviving Sepsis Campaign Bundles

To be completed within 3 hours:
1. Measure lactate level
2. Obtain blood cultures prior to administration of antibiotics
3. Administer broad spectrum antibiotics
4. Administer 30 mL/kg crystalloid for hypotension or lactate ≥4 mmol/L

To be completed within 6 hours:
5. Apply vasopressors (for hypotension that does not respond to initial fluid resuscitation) to maintain a mean arterial pressure (MAP) ≥65 mm Hg
6. In the event of persistent arterial hypotension despite volume resuscitation (septic shock) or initial lactate ≥4 mmol/L (36 mg/dL):
   – Measure central venous pressure (CVP)*
   – Measure central venous oxygen saturation (ScvO$_2$)*
7. Remeasure lactate if initial lactate was elevated*

* Targets for quantitative resuscitation included in the guidelines are CVP of ≥8 mm Hg; ScvO$_2$ of ≥70%, and normalization of lactate.

Cardiogenic Shock

Cardiogenic shock is inadequate tissue perfusion resulting from primary heart problem due to myocardial or valvular dysfunction. It presents with hypotension, cool peripheries, distended neck veins, oliguria, altered mental status and respiratory failure due to pulmonary edema. Central venous pressures may be elevated with high systemic vascular resistance and reduced cardiac index.

Causes

- Myocardial infarction
- Left ventricular failure
- Cardiomyopathy
- Valvular abnormalities
- Trauma.

This should be differentiated from other forms of shock.

Management

Identify and try to treat the cause if possible. For myocardial infarction, reperfusion therapy should be instituted as soon as possible. Patients might need fluids depending on the volume status and in right ventricular infarction. Pulmonary artery floatation catheter may be useful in guiding fluid therapy. Dobutamine may be used for its inodilator effects as can phosphodiesterase inhibitors like milrinone/enoximone and levosimendan. Dopamine and noradrenaline may be used for resistant hypotension cautiously. Vasodilators are preferred if blood pressure is more stable. Diuretics used in pulmonary edema along with non-invasive ventilation to offload the heart. Intra-aortic balloon pump and emergency PCI/CABG are used in refractory cases. Patients with either recoverable ventricular failures or awaiting transplantation may be put on left or right ventricular assist devices (LVAD/RVAD) and extracorporeal membrane oxygenators (ECMO).

Hypovolemic Shock

Hypovolemia is a result of decreased circulating blood volume resulting in end organ dysfunction or damage. This is also associated with salt depletion, hence different from dehydration where predominantly free water is lost. It presents with hypotension, cool peripheries, collapsed veins, poor capillary refill time and organ dysfunctions like acute kidney injury with oliguria, tachycardia, tachypnea and altered mental state.

Causes

- Trauma and bleeding
- Diarrhea and vomiting
- Severe burns
- Surgical blood loss
- Heat stroke
- Fasting.

This should be differentiated from other causes of shock.

Stages of Shock

Table 8.1: Stages of shock and recommendation on fluid therapy

Blood loss	<750	750–1500	1500–2000	>2000
Blood loss (%bw)	<15%	15–30%	3–40%	>40%
Pulse	<100	100–120	120–140	>140
BP	>100	>100	<100	<100
Pulse volume	Normal	↓	↓	↓
Respiration rate	14–20	20–30	30–35	>35
Hourly urine output	>30	20–30	<20	<20
Mental status	Marked anxiety	Mild anxiety	Anxiety/confusion	Confusion/drowsiness
Fluid therapy	Crystalloids	Crystalloids	Crystalloids/colloids/blood	Crystalloids/colloid/blood

Management

Rapid recognition is essential for the management of this condition. If treatment with fluids is started early, all abnormalities can be corrected early. Assess the airway and breathing followed by estimation and restoration of fluids. Blood and colloids are used appropriately depending on the blood loss and volume status. Vital parameters are checked regularly to see the response and adequacy of resuscitation. Surgical advice should be sought early to find source of bleeding and control.

Obstructive Shock

Extracardiac obstruction to blood flow can lead to obstructive shock where the effective circulatory flow is limited. It can present like cardiogenic shock with hypotension, tachycardia, cool peripheries, distended neck veins, pulsus paradoxus, reduced heart sounds, renal injury and altered mentation. ECG may show tachycardia and reduced amplitude.

Causes

- Impaired diastolic filling (reduced preload)
    - Direct venous obstruction (vena caval obstruction) due to intrathoracic tumors
    - Increased intrathoracic pressure
        - Tension pneumothorax
        - Mechanical ventilation with excess pressure
        - Asthma

- Decreased cardiac compliance
  - Constrictive pericarditis
  - Cardiac tamponade
- ❑ Impaired systolic contraction (increased afterload)
  - Right ventricle
    - Pulmonary embolus
    - Acute pulmonary hypertension
  - Left ventricle
    - Saddle embolus
    - Aortic dissection (rarely).

Diagnosis starts with suspicion of the disorder. CXR can diagnose pneumothorax and pulmonary embolus in some cases. Echocardiogram will diagnose tamponade and right heart strain in pulmonary embolism. The tamponade may be due to infection (tuberculosis), uremia, trauma, malignancy, or idiopathic. This should be differentiated from constrictive pericarditis, restrictive cardiomyopathy, left ventricular failure and right ventricular failure.

Management

Once the problem is diagnosed, treatment should be instituted appropriately. Fluids should be used with caution. Many of the disorders are life threatening if not treated immediately. For tension pneumothorax, needle thoracotomy followed by intercostal drain insertion can immediately improve the hemodynamics. PE can be treated with thrombolysis and cardiac tamponade as described previously. Surgical consult should be obtained as soon as possible in appropriate cases.

Neurogenic Shock

Neurogenic shock is a type of distributive shock causing hypotension along with bradycardia. This is because of autonomic system failure resulting from injury to the spinal cord. This leads to a reduction in sympathetic tone in the blood vessels with pooling of blood in the peripheries. If the injury is above T6, loss of thoracic sympathetic tone leads to bradycardia with hypotension; whereas if the injury is lower, unopposed sympathetic tone will cause tachycardia and increase contractility. The extremities are warm above and cold below the level of injury. Hypotension will be profound and occasionally resistant to treatment. This should be differentiated from other causes of shock.

Causes

- ❑ Brain injury
- ❑ Cervical or high thoracic spinal injury.

Management

The site of injury should be investigated. Fluids are the initial treatment of such spinal shock. Fluid resuscitation may be followed by vasopressor support in selected cases with noradrenaline or dopamine. Vasopressin can also be used in resistant cases. If bradycardia persists, atropine can be used too. Ventilatory support may be required if the injury is higher and spine stabilization is necessary in such cases.

Anaphylactic Shock

Anaphylactic reaction is a IgE mediated allergic reaction which can lead to shock and death if not recognized and treated immediately. The symptoms include rash, throat swelling, wheezing and hypotension commonly. It appears in about 5–30 minutes after exposure though this can lag by several hours. This results in sudden release of immunological mediators from mast cells and basophils. This causes a general system affection leading to rashes, angiedema, bronchospasm, tachycardia, hypotension, arrhythmia, cramps, diarrhea, seizures and coma. This can be triggered by foods like peanuts and fish, medications, venoms, latex, aspirin, radiocontrast, and antibiotics amongst other things. If the following symptoms develop within minutes of exposure to an allergen, there is high likelihood of anaphylaxis:

- Involvement of skin or mucosal surface
- Respiratory difficulties
- Cardiovascular collapse
- GI symptoms.

This should be differentiated from cardiogenic shock, sepsis, poisoning and epilepsy.

Types

- *Anaphylactic shock*: Occurs within minutes of exposure to the allergen
- *Delayed anaphylaxis*: Occurs up to days after the initial exposure. Has the same mechanism and treated in the same way
- *Anaphylactoid reactions*: Occur due to mast cell degranulation and does not involve the allergy pathway.

Management

Assess and manage airway and breathing. Intubation and ventilation may be need in severe cases. IV fluids are required for volume expansion. Adrenaline should be used in suspected cases as soon as possible in the dose of 0.3–0.5 mg IM or 0.1 mg IV in repeated doses titrated to effect. Histamine antagonists are used alongside to block H1 and H2 receptors (chlorpheniramine and ranitidine commonly). Steroids are also used for late reactions. Vasopressors may need to be used. Tryptase levels can be send to diagnose mast cell degranulation. If it is recognized early and treated appropriately, it has a very good prognosis.

Suggested Reading

1. Brown SG, Mullins RJ, Gold MS. Anaphylaxis: diagnosis and management. The Medical Journal of Australia. 2006;185(5):283-9.
2. Guly HR, Bouamra O, Lecky FE. The incidence of neurogenic shock in patients with isolated spinal cord injury in the emergency department. Resuscitation. 2008; 76:57-62.
3. Maier RV. Approach to the patient with shock. In: Fauci As, Harrison TR, (Eds.). Harrison's Principles of Internal Medicine. 17th Ed. New York, NY: McGraw Hill; 2008:Chap 264.
4. Saraswat N, Hollenberg SM. Cardiogenic shock. Hospital Practice. 2010;38(1):74-83.
5. Surviving sepsis campaign: International guidelines for management of severe sepsis and septic shock: 2012. http://www.sccm.org/Documents/SSCGuidelines. pdf - accessed May 15, 2014.

CHAPTER 9

Endocrine Problems in ICU

Diabetic Ketoacidosis

Diabetic ketoacidosis is a life-threatening emergency in patients with diabetes mellitus, predominantly seen in patients with type 1 diabetes. This results from lack of insulin, when the body starts metabolizing fat for its energy needs producing ketone bodies in the process.

The clinical presentation is with polyuria, polydipsia, abdominal pain, vomiting, fatigue, lethargy and coma. There will be marked dehydration, tachycardia, hypotension, tachypnea due to acidosis and fruity odor in the breath. This can be precipitated by infection, missed insulin dose, myocardial infarction or angina, medications, pancreatitis and other stressors. The lack of insulin and/or an excess glucagon leads to breakdown of glycogen to glucose leading to hyperglycemia. This in turn leads to glycosuria and osmotic diuresis with it. Exaggerated diabetes symptoms are seen because of this with polydipsia, polyuria and dehydration. Lack of insulin in the peripheral tissues leads to breakdown of fat into fatty acids to form ketone bodies (acetoacetate and beta-hydroxybutyrate) resulting in acidosis and its effects.

Diagnosis

Hyperglycemia, ketones in blood or urine and acidosis are classical findings in diabetic ketoacidosis (DKA). Arterial blood gas analysis will show acidosis with compensatory respiratory alkalosis. Electrolytes and renal function tests (urea nitrogen and creatinine) should be measured along with investigations for the cause for the precipitation of DKA.

It can be divided into:
- Mild: pH between 7.25–7.30
- Moderate: pH between 7.00–7.25
- Severe: pH<7.00.

Management

Fluid replacement remains the mainstay of treatment due to severe dehydration associated with DK. Normal saline (0.9% NaCl) remains the fluid of choice. Insulin is essential too to stop the peripheral ketosis and fat metabolism and reduce the formation of ketoacids. Bolus dose of 0.1 unit per kg is sometimes administered followed by an infusion at the rate of 0.1 unit/kg/h. Once the blood glucose starts coming down, the rate can be reduced or glucose drip added.

With the addition of insulin, care should be taken at the electrolyte levels as insulin will drive the potassium into the cells leading to dangerous hypokalemia. Potassium should hence be measured regularly and replaced in the IV fluids. Close monitoring is essential with regular blood glucose and electrolytes. Caution should be exercised if there is associated cardiac and renal dysfunction. Treatment of the precipitating cause should undertaken along with the DKA. If the neurological function worsens with treatment, ICU admission is warranted and fluids should be managed carefully. This may mean cerebral edema which can be fatal if not managed appropriately.

Hyperosmolar Non-ketotic Diabetic Coma

Hyperosmolar non-ketotic coma (HONK) or hyperosmolar hyperglycemic state (HHS) occurs when the blood sugars rise to dangerously high levels causing increased osmolarity and dehydration. This is more commonly seen in type 2 diabetics with low or no detectable ketones. It carries a higher morbidity and mortality than diabetic ketocidosis (DKA). This is generally associated with altered mental status and can be precipitated by infection, stroke, angina or myocardial infarction, or other acute illnesses. There is a relative insulin deficiency leading to polyuria, dehydration and hemoconcentration. There is still some insulin present, preventing the ketosis that is seen in DKA.

Diagnosis

American Diabetes Association has published guidance on the diagnosis of HONK:
1. Plasma glucose >600 mg/dL
2. Serum osmolality >320 mOsm/kg
3. Profound dehydration needing up to 9 L fluid replacement
4. Serum pH >7.30
5. Bicarbonate >15 mEq/L
6. Small or absent ketonuria/ketonemia
7. Alteration in conciousness.

This is seen more with elderly patients, reduced intake, sepsis, and obese patients.

Management

Aggressive fluid resuscitation is required with isotonic solutions. Preferred IV fluid is normal saline. Caution should be exercised as a big proportion of patients are elderly with underlying cardiac and renal dysfunction. The fluids should be replaced over 24–48 hours. Small amount of insulin will be required, but caution as blood glucose reduces rapidly with fluid replacement. Replace electrolytes and careful monitoring required to avoid cerebral edema. Identification of the cause of deterioration and treatment of the cause should be carried along with HONK treatment.

Hypoglycemia

Hypoglycemia is a life-threatening medical emergency involving a dangerously low blood glucose. This can present as seizures, confusion, dysphoria, coma and rarely permanent brain damage or death. This commonly is seen in patients who have diabetes mellitus and are on treatment. It is rarely seen in other group of patients including patients having insulinomas, alcoholics, adrenal failure, prolonged starvation, inborn error of metabolisms, severe infections, liver failure and poisoning. Apart from the effects on brain, autonomic effects can also be seen like diaphoresis, palpitations, anxiety, nausea, hunger, visual disturbances and weakness.

Diagnosis

Whipple's triad is generally used for diagnosis. This includes:
1. Symptoms of hypoglycemia
2. Low blood sugar
3. Resolution of symptoms with glucose treatment.

Blood sugars are generally maintained between 72–144 mg/dL. Symptoms of hypoglycemia generally occur below 50–55 mg/dL levels. Differentiate from myxedema coma, delirium, sepsis, pheochromocytoma, inadvertent overdose, suicide attempts, liver failure and neurosis. Significant episodes of hypoglycemia can increase the risk of cardiac events.

Management

If patient awake, glucose containing fluids can be given orally. Other food products like biscuits, orange, apple or juices can also be used given orally. The effects start within 5 minutes and full symptom resolution should be expected in 10–20 minutes. If the patients are combative or comatosed, intravenous route can be used. IV dextrose can then be infused and patients should respond pretty quickly. IM glucagon can be used in cases where IV access is difficult or not possible.

Adrenal Failure

Adrenal insufficiency results from a relative lack of adrenal hormones including steroids like cortisol and mineralocorticoids like aldosterone. Adrenal insufficiency presents as severe abdominal cramps, weakness, nausea, vomiting, hypotension, hypovolemia with vasoplegia, altered mentation and confusion. Adrenal crisis occurs when body is subject to stress like infection, trauma, injury or surgery and if left untreated, can result in death.

It can be divided into:
1. *Primary*: due to direct impairment of adrenal glands due to autoimmune disease (Addison's disease), idiopathic or congenital causes.
2. *Secondary*: due to decreased release of adrenocorticotropic hormone (ACTH) from the pituitary mainly due to exogenous use of steroids leading to suppression of hypothalamic pituitary adrenal (HPA) axis. Pituitary adenoma may cause the same effect as can Sheehan's syndrome.
3. *Tertiary*: due to hypothalamic disorder leading to decreased corticotropin releasing hormone (CRH).

Hyper pigmentation may result if primary adrenal failure present with increased ACTH. Hyponatremia, hyperkalemia, hypoglycemia, renal failure, and hypercalcemia are present often in such cases.

Diagnosis

Serum cortisol is usually <20 μg/dL and ACTH stimulation test increment of cortisol >7 μg/dL or peak cortisol >17 μg/dL excludes diagnosis. There is low or absent cortisol, increased ACTH and abnormal stimulation in primary hypoaldosteronism. Anyone on long-term steroids equivalent to 30 mg/day of hydrocortisone will have relative adrenal insufficiency. Secondary adrenal insufficiency may be due to pituitary or hypothalamic causes where ACTH is low and MRI may be needed to diagnose the cause.

Management

During adrenal crisis, intravenous fluids should be started and intravenous steroids should be given as soon as possible. If ACTH test is planned, dexamethasone can be used as it doesn't interfere with the steroid measurements, but therapy should not be delayed for the test. If primary steroid deficiency is detected, any of the steroids can be used including dexamethasone, prednisolone, methylprednisolone, hydrocortisone or prednisone; whereas if mineralocorticoid deficiency is detected, fludrocortisone can be used. Electrolytes should be corrected, and glucose should be monitored. May need vasopressor support along with treatment of the cause.

Cushing's Syndrome

Cushing's syndrome is a set of signs and symptoms associated with exposure to steroids. This can be due to treatment with steroids or inherent high production of cortisol in the body.

Cushing's syndrome presents with weakness, weight gain, hirsutism, irregular menses, moon facies, buffalo hump, easy bruising, central obesity, diabetes, hypertension, increased lipids, increased risk of cardiac problems, osteoporosis, hyperglycemia, hypokalemia, and metabolic alkalosis. All this is a result of high levels of cortisol or steroids in the body.

The most common cause for Cushing's syndrome is exogenous steroids to treat diseases like asthma, rheumatoid arthritis and other autoimmune disorders. The adrenals atrophy in these cases.

Endogenous Cushing's syndrome results from:
1. Pituitary adenoma: leading to adrenocorticotropic hormone (ACTH) excess and increased adrenal steroids (Cushing's disease)
2. Adrenal Cushing's: from adrenal adenoma or hyperplasia
3. ACTH producing tumors: leading to paraneoplastic Cushing's syndrome.

Diagnosis

Cortisol levels are increased and low dose dexamethasone doesn't suppress cortisol levels. ACTH levels are raised in pituitary disease and high dose dexamethasone test may be required to rule out abnormal ACTH release. MRI may be needed. Differentiate from diabetes mellitus, obesity, depression and drug induced Cushing's syndrome. Cushing's disease is Cushing's syndrome due to pituitary cause (increased secretion of ACTH).

Management

Iatrogenic Cushing's syndrome will need replacing the steroids with other drugs or slowly cutting down the steroids to a minimum. Surgical correction may be needed in adrenal tumor, pituitary adenoma, or other tumors secreting ACTH. Refractory adrenal hyperplasia may need bilateral adrenalectomies. Medical management is needed in some cases where surgery is not possible or refused by the patient. Ketoconazole or metyrapone have been shown to inhibit cortisol synthesis. Mifepristone can be used for cognitive dysfunction seen with Cushing's syndrome.

Thyrotoxicosis

Hyperthyroidism results from increased secretion of thyroid hormones leading to hypermetabolism in the body and the subsequent signs and symptoms that include nervousness, increased appetite, sweating, weight loss, weakness, confusion, agitation and coma. Temperature regulation is altered and tachycardia, arrhythmia, hypertension, heart failure, opthalmopathy, tremor, myopathy and cachexia may result. Goiter may be present. Sometimes this results from inflammation of the thyroid gland (thyroiditis) or exogenous thyroid ingestion. The majority are caused by Grave's disease (autoimmune disease). Toxic adenoma and toxic multinodular goiter account for most of the other cases though drugs, thyroiditis, teratoma or pituitary adenoma may also be responsible. Thyroid storm may be precipitated in uncontrolled cases due to any stress including myocardial infarction, sepsis, surgery, stroke, trauma and anesthesia which can be life threatening. This should be differentiated from sepsis, overdose, withdrawal from alcohol, and pheochromocytoma.

Diagnosis

Laboratory tests will reveal increased T4 and T3, with depressed TSH. This may be associated with increased bilirubin, alkaline phosphatase, calcium and AST. Specific antibodies are found in Grave's disease (anti-TSH receptor antibodies) and Hashimoto's thyroiditis (anti-thyroid peroxidase antibodies). Thyroid scans and radio-iodine uptake studies may be carried out to distinguish the causes.

Management

Identify and treat the precipitating cause. Propylthiouracil and methimazole are used to reduce hormone synthesis and peripheral T4 to T3 conversion. Iodine can be used to reduce release of thyroxin into circulation. Systemic effects are reduced by non-specific beta-blockers like propranolol. Variables like blood pressure, temperature, fluid and electrolyte disturbances are similarly corrected. Steroids may be useful if adrenal insufficiency suspected. Surgery is not used extensively as most causes can be treated with medical therapy. Thyroid storms are treated with fluid management along with beta-blockers and anti-thyroid drugs like methimazole and intravenous steroids.

Myxedema due to Hypothyroidism

Myxedema or severe hypothyroidism occurs due to relative lack of thyroid hormones. It represents the skin manifestations of hypothyroidism (occasionally seen in hyperthyroidism too!). The patients present with cold intolerance, weight gain, constipation, depression, puffy face, dry, rough and cold skin, hair loss, large tongue, hypothermia, bradycardia, hypoxia and respiratory failure, confusion, sleepiness and coma. There is deposition of mucopolysaccharides in the dermis resulting in swelling.

Diagnosis

Bloods will reveal low T4 and T3 and elevated TSH. Hypoglycaemia, hyponatremia, anemia, increased creatine kinase (CK), creatinine and hyperlipidemia may be present. Many patients may present with hypothermia. ECG will reveal bradycardia with non-specific ST-T changes, prolonged QT and blocks. Most often this presents in known hypothyroid patients under stress or missed medications. This should be differentiated from hypothermia, poisoning, obstructive sleep apnea (OSA), Parkinsonism, etc.

Management

Immediate replacement of thyroid hormones is essential to reverse this condition. Oral thyroxin or intravenous tri-iodo thyronine are used in these cases. Intravenous steroids are required if adrenal insufficiency present to prevent Addisonian crisis when metabolic rate increases. Correct hypovolemia and electrolyte abnormalities. For reduced consciousness and respiratory failure, ventilatory support may be required. Identify and treat precipitating cause.

Suggested Reading

1. Cryer PE, Axelrod L, Grossman AB, Heller SR, Montori VM, Seaquist ER, et al. "Evaluation and management of adult hypoglycemic disorders: an Endocrine Society Clinical Practice Guideline". J Clin Endocrinol Metab. 2009;94(3):709-28.
2. Eledrisi MS, Alshanti MS, Shah MF, Brolosy B, Jaha N. "Overview of the diagnosis and management of diabetic ketoacidosis". American Journal of Medical Science. 2006;331(5):243-51.
3. Nieman LK, Ilias I. "Evaluation and treatment of Cushing's syndrome." The American Journal of Medicine. 2005;118(12):1340-6.
4. Siraj, Elias S. "Update on the Diagnosis and Treatment of Hyperthyroidism". Journal of Clinical Outcomes Management. 2008;15(6):298-307
5. Stoner, GD. "Hyperosmolar hyperglycemic state". American Family Physician. 2005;71(9):1723-30.
6. Ten S, New M, Maclaren N. "Clinical review 130: Addison's disease 2001". J Clin Endocrinol Metab. 2001;86(7):2909-22.

CHAPTER 10

Oncological Emergencies

Acute Leukemia

Acute leukemia occurs when hematopoietic cells transform malignantly into primitive cells. They can be myelocytic or lymphocytic and replace the normal bone marrow tissue causing anemia, thrombocytopenia and granulocytopenia. Other organs can be infiltrated like liver, spleen, lymph nodes, kidney and gonads. The patients generally describe weakness and lethargy due to anemia, repeated infections due to low white cell count (WCC) and bleeding due to thrombocytopenia. Examination may be normal, but fever, pallor, petechiae, hemorrhages, lymphadenopathy, splenomegaly may be present. Blood smear may show increased WCC, thrombocytopenia and blast cells. Auer rods distinguish lymphoblastic from myeloblastic leukemia. Chemical markers and cytogenetics are required for prognostication and treatment options. Bone marrow examintation is used to confirm the type and presence of leukemia. Acute myeloid leukemia (AML) has 7 subtypes and acute promyelocytic leukemia is associated with disseminated intravascular coagulation (DIC) and spontaneous hemorrhage. Differentiate from aplastic anemia, leukemoid reaction and tumor infiltration.

Management

Prognosis has improved in the recent years with the availability of new drugs. It remains guarded in infants and elderly patients and patients with involvement of organs like kidneys, liver and spleen. Chemotherapy is the basis of treatment for most of leukemias. This may be followed by bone marrow suppression and may require long-term transfusion to correct the deficit. Infection control measures are essential and long-term catheters may be required for infusion of chemotherapeautic agents. Antibiotics may be required for leukopenia and tumor lysis syndrome may result with chemotherapy (discussed later). Acute promyelocytic leukemia responds to all-trans retinoic acid (ATRA). Selected patients benefit from bone marrow transplant.

Golden Tips

- AML is the most common acute leukemia in adults
- Chemotherapy is used to prolong survival in most types of leukemias

- Stem cell transplant has been used with success in young and resistant cases.

Tumor Lysis Syndrome

Tumor lysis is a metabolic syndrome occurring due to rapid destruction of cells due to chemotherapy in some leukemias. This can sometimes happen spontaneously in lymphomas or some leukemias without any chemotherapy. This can lead to hyperkalemia, hyperphosphatemia, and hyperuricemia with resultant hypocalcemia. Renal failure may result from uric acid and stone formation. ECG changes, arrhythmias, convulsions, tetany, cramps and malaise results. More often seen in solid tumors with rapid destruction of cells.

Diagnosis

Cairo and Bishop have defined classification for the tumor lysis syndrome
- Laboratory tumor lysis syndrome:
  - Uric acid >8 mg/dL
  - Potassium >6 mEq/L
  - Phosphate >4.5 mg/dL
  - Calcium <7 mg/dL.
- Clinical tumor lysis syndrome
  - Increase in serum creatinine (>1.5 times upper limit of normal)
  - Cardiac arrhythmias or sudden death
  - Seizure disorder.

Management

- Aggressive volume loading is required to flush the electrolytes and uric acid in the urine
- Allopurinol before chemotherapy may prevent some of the complications
- Hyperkalemia needs appropriate treatment as this can be fatal
- Alkalinization of urine may be required with hyperuricemia
- Occasional renal replacement therapy in the form of dialysis is required for life-threatening electrolyte abnormalities.

Superior Vena Cava Syndrome

Superior vena cava syndrome results from compression, invasion or thrombosis of the superior vena cava commonly due to malignancy. The most common malignancy is the bronchogenic carcinoma. The venous return from the upper body is hence hampered leading to venous stagnation.

Symptoms

The symptoms resulting from this are:
- Upper body fullness
- Headache and cough

- Dizziness
- Venous distension
- Plethora on the face and cyanosis
- Edema
- Dyspnea because of airway compromise.

Diagnosis is essentially clinical and supported/confirmed by CXR, CT scan and later tissue biopsy. CXR will show mediastinal widening, while CT scans will show the underlying cause and the extent of the disease. Common malignancies are lymphoma, lung cancer, aneurysms, tuberculosis, infection, thrombosis of veins, etc. This should be differentiated from angioedema, goiter, and DVT of upper extremity.

Management

- Glucocorticoids are used to reduce the inflammation and edema in the surrounding tissue to improve venous drainage
- Tumors like lymphoma are steroid responsive and sometimes lead to complete resolution of symptoms
- Diuretics are used to reduce the venous congestion
- Endovascular stenting may be tried in the interim
- Depending on the cause, surgical techniques are used for acute relief and radiotherapy in cases where surgery is not feasible
- Chemotherapy treatment of choice for small lung cell cancer, lymphoma and germ cell tumors
- Head end should be elevated and oxygen administered if required
- The mortality is often related to the tumor rather than the obstruction.

Suggested Reading

1. Davidson MB, Thakkar S, Hix JK, et al. Pathophysiology, clinical consequences and treatment of tumor lysis syndrome. Am J Med. 2003;116(8):546-54.
2. Guidance on haematological cancers from National Institute for Clinical Excellence (UK): http://www.nice.org.uk/nicemedia/live/10891/28786/28786.pdf Accessed June 2014.
3. Rice TW, Rodriquez RM, Light RW. The superior vena cava syndrome: clinical characteristics and evolving etiology. Medicine. 2006;85(1):37-42.

CHAPTER 11

Pregnancy and ICU

Preeclampsia and Eclampsia

Preeclampsia and eclampsia are diseases of pregnancy associated with dysregulation of vasomotor tone. Preeclampsia presents with hypertension, proteinuria and edema; although edema has been omitted now from the diagnosis since this is present in most pregnant population. Severe preeclampsia is defined as blood pressure >160/110 mm Hg, more proteinuria, increased creatinine, pulmonary edema, oliguria, liver dysfunction and intrauterine growth retardation. Eclampsia is defined as presence of seizures. This can be complicated by HELLP syndrome (**h**emolysis, **e**levated **l**iver enzymes and **l**ow **p**latelets). Preeclampsia generally occurs in previously normotensive patients or hypertensive patients after 20 weeks of gestation and has higher incidence in multiple pregnancies or hydatidiform mole. Differentials include chronic hypertension, acute fatty liver of pregnancy, and chronic renal disease.

Treatment

Definitive treatment is delivery of fetus.

Seizures should be controlled with magnesium sulfate with the therapeutic range of 4.8–8.4 mg/dL with repeated deep tendon reflexes examination. Blood pressure should be controlled with hydralazine and labetalol, occasionally sodium nitroprusside may need to be used. Urine output monitoring is essential. Fluids should be restricted as pulmonary edema may result from fluid overload. Central venous pressure monitoring may be needed in selected patients to guide fluid therapy. ICU stay is needed in patients who have difficult to control hypertension, have end organ damage or present with seizures. Control of airway may become essential occasionally. Caution is advised due to airway edema and pregnant state that may lead to aspiration risk. Delivery of fetus should be carried out as soon as practically feasible, but the reversal of preeclampsia is only noticed after a few days and patients may even worsen after delivery.

Acute Fatty Liver of Pregnancy

Fatty infiltration in pregnancy can occur rapidly with deterioration of liver function. This may present with nausea, vomiting, pain, anorexia and malaise. This occurs mostly in the last trimester or post-delivery and is associated with raised alanine transaminase (ALT), aspartate aminotransferase (AST), alkaline phosphatase, bilirubin, white cell count, coagulopathy, occasional disseminated intravascular coagulation (DIC) and hypoglycemia. This may later progress to hepatic necrosis, fulminant hepatic failure, renal failure, cerebral edema, fetal loss, pancreatitis and hypoglycemia. This should be differentiated from preeclampsia, hepatic rupture, cholecystitis, HELLP syndrome and drug-induced liver dysfunction.

Management

Continuous fetal monitoring is essential. Vitals including neurological examination is important. Correct fluid and electrolyte imbalances, glucose containing solutions may be required along with blood products. Fetus should be delivered as soon as patient stable and this is soon followed by correction of liver dysfunction. Vitamin K, lactulose and nutrition should be part of the management. Liver transplant may occasionally be required in severe fulminant hepatic necrosis.

Amniotic Fluid Embolism

Amniotic fluid embolism is a rare obstetric emergency where amniotic fluid, fetal cells and other debris come in contact with the maternal circulation leading to a catastrophic allergic reaction. This can result during spontaneous labor, vaginal or cesarean section delivery or following termination of pregnancy. The reaction presents as sudden cardiorespiratory collapse leading to hypotension, dyspnea and wheezing. Seizures, disseminated intravascular coagulation (DIC), acute respiratory distress syndrome (ARDS) like features may also be present. Echocardiography (ECHO) will reveal left ventricular dysfunction along with pulmonary hypertension. It is seen in 1:8000 to 1:80000 deliveries worldwide and there is often poor reporting due to lack of specific diagnostic tools. The fist phase is the phase of circulatory collapse and has high mortality close to 50%. If the patients survive this, the second phase is manifested in the form of coagulopathy or DIC. Many are left with neurological consequences. Differentials include pulmonary embolism, sepsis, air embolism, myocardial infarction, anaphylaxis or other adverse reaction to drugs.

Management

Oxygenation and ventilation are paramount. There is no specific treatment for amniotic fluid embolism and supportive measures are used for cardiovascular collapse. Many of the symptoms are caused by release of serotonin, thromboxane and vagal stimulation. A combination of ondansetron, metoclopramide, atropine and ketorolac along with other supportive measures are used in many cases with good results. Circulatory support in the form of vasopressors and inotropes may be required and central venous access may be needed. Correct fluid and electrolyte imbalance along with coagulopathy. Deliver the fetus as soon as possible to increase likelihood of successful resuscitation.

Septic Abortion

Septic abortion results from a miscarriage associated with uterine infection. This can occur after spontaneous or induced termination of pregnancy. It presents with vaginal discharge, pain within 7 days of termination or instrumentation of uterus. This can rapidly lead to shock and hemorrhage. The other presenting features may be chills and fever, severe abdominal pain, heavy and prolonged vaginal bleeding, foul discharge and backache. Peritonism may be present depending on extent of infection spread. This may progress to signs of septic shock with hypotension, hypothermia or pyrexia, oliguria and altered mentation. The risk factors for septic abortion are retained intrauterine device (IUD), ruptured membranes, sexually transmitted diseases (STDs), unsafe abortion practices and insertion of foreign bodies. Products of conception may still be present. Cultures should be obtained and commonly polymicrobial infections are present including aerobic and anaerobic bacteria. This can occasionally be associated with perforations of uterus and bowel. Prognosis is poor if gas-forming organisms are present or patient presents very late in septic shock. This should be differentiated from perforations, puerperal sepsis and septic shock from prolonged rupture of membranes.

Management

Full examination with cultures of the discharge is important. Prompt fluid resuscitation with intravenous fluids and antibiotics should be started. Many patients will need surgical intervention to remove products of conception and debride the uterus. Radical surgeries like hysterectomy may be needed in severe infections also involving the fallopian tubes and ovaries.

Pregnancy and Asthma

Asthma is the most common medical condition during pregnancy. The presentation is similar with dyspnea, chest tightness and wheeze. Accessory muscle use, tachypnea and tachycardia will be associated. Asthma will remain stable in 1/3rd, worsens in 1/3rd and improves in 1/3rd. The signs and symptoms depend on the compliance with treatment. The clinical symptoms generally worsen during the 2nd trimester and can improve as pregnancy progresses. Generally asthma will not affect labor and delivery.

Investigations

Pulmonary function tests should be done with each visit. During acute attack, arterial gases may show hypoxia, but low $paCO_2$ may be present physiologically due to pregnancy; hence normal $paCO_2$ may be an early sign of fatigue. Compliance with treatment is essential. Confirm history and hospital admissions including ICU admissions. Prolonged hypoxia may adversely affect the fetus. Differentiate from congestive cardiac failure, pulmonary emboli, pneumothorax and pneumonia.

Management

Acute attacks are managed as a normal asthmatic. Regular spirometry may show response to treatment. Beta agonists used as first line treatment. Oral steroids are considered for acute attack followed by inhaled steroids for control. Supplemental oxygen is given to keep saturations normal. Antibiotics may be considered if suspicion of bacterial infections. Mechanical ventilation may be needed in severe cases. Most medications including theophylline, leukotriene antatonists and steroids have been used for a long time in pregnant patients without significant increase in fetal defects. Caution though should still be exercised for all medications and the minimum treatment required should be used without compromising the control of symptoms.

Pulmonary Edema in Pregnancy

Pulmonary edema in pregnancy is a life-threatening complication during pregnancy. It presents with dyspnea, cough, chest tightness, frothy sputum and hypoxia. Bilateral crepitations may be present along with tachycardia and tachypnea. CXR will reveal congestion and occasional pleural effusions. This can occur without any predisposing condition in pregnancy; but the risk increases if hypertension, structural heart defects, overload, or cardiomyopathy are present. Increased cardiac output, increased extracellular fluid, decreased oncotic pressure and fluids in pregnancy increase the chance of development of pulmonary edema. The patients are more predisposed during preeclampsia.

Investigations

Apart from CXR for diagnosis, echocardiography is indicated for structural defects, cardiomyopathy, and valvular heart disease. Cardiogenic pulmonary edema may also occur in acute coronary syndromes and cardiac enzymes are hence indicated. This should be differentiated from pulmonary embolism, myocardial ischemia, cardiomyopathy, asthma and pneumonia.

Management

Dramatic improvement should be seen with treatment. Fluids should be restricted and tocolytic agents discontinued if possible. Diuretics and oxygen are the mainstay of treatment. Antibiotics may be needed if infection is associated. Continuous fetal monitoring is needed. If there is delay in resolution of symptoms, consider secondary causes and structural problems which should be seen in echocardiography. ICU admission is generally needed for close monitoring and treatment. In the presence of valvular disease, cardiology or cardiothoracic services may need to evaluate regarding intervention.

Suggested Reading

1. Figueroa MS, Peters JI. Congestive heart failure: Diagnosis, pathophysiology, therapy, and implications for respiratory care. Respir Care. 2006;51(4):403-12.
2. Riely CA. Acute fatty liver of pregnancy. Semin Liver Dis. 1987;7(1):47-54.
3. Schatz M, Dombrowski MP. Clinical practice. Asthma in pregnancy. N Engl J Med. 2009; 360:1862.
4. Stafford I, Sheffield J. Amniotic fluid embolism. Obstet Gynecol Clin North Am. 2007;34(3):545-53, xii.
5. Steegers EAP, von Dadelszen P, Duvekot JJ, Pijnenborg R. Preeclampsia. Lancet. 2010;376(9741):631-44.
6. Stubblefield PF, Grimes DA. Septic abortion. NEJM. 1994;331:310-4.

CHAPTER 12

Gastrointestinal Diseases

Small Bowel Obstruction

Diagnosis and Presentation

This presents with intermittent colicky abdominal pain and constipation, bloating, nausea and vomiting. Tenderness, distension, active peristalsis associated with pain. There will be associated fluid depletion and electrolyte abnormalities. Distended bowel loops will be visible on X-rays along with ladder like patters and air fluid levels (Fig. 12.1). Thumb printing and presence of gas in bowel wall suggest necrosis. CT may reveal the site of obstruction. This may be due to adhesions, tumors, hernias, volvulus, radiotherapy, etc. Aspiration pneumonia, strangulation, infarction, sepsis, perforation may all result if this is not treated. Differentiate from paralytic ileus, large bowel obstruction, ascites, pancreatitis, inflammatory bowel disease and appendicitis.

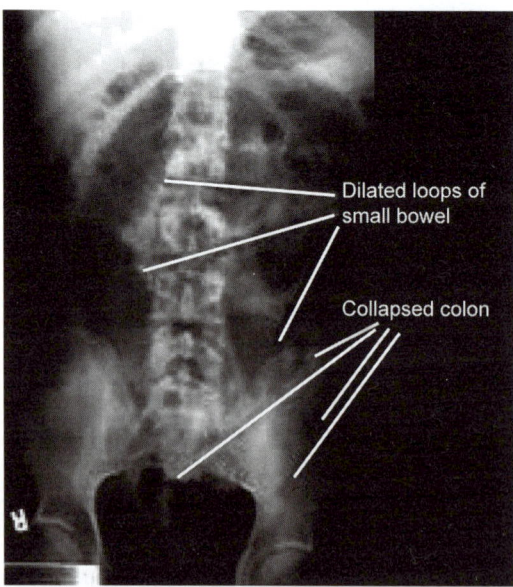

FIGURE 12.1: Typical abdominal X-ray in acute small bowel obstruction

Management

Bowel obstruction may present as an emergency with septic shock. Active resuscitation with fluids and electrolyte correction is needed. Nasogastric tube to decompress the stomach and small bowel may be needed and the fluids replaced accordingly. Central venous line and arterial lines are often needed for hemodynamic monitoring and fluid replacement. Surgical advise is sought early and may need emergent surgery depending on the patients condition and pathology. Broad spectrum antibiotics are usually started and cultures sent as needed. Multiple organ failure can develop and can lead to fatality. Often serum lactates may be elevated.

Large Bowel Obstruction

Diagnosis and Presentation

Large bowel obstruction presents with constipation and cramping pain. Vomiting is a late finding and may not occur at all. Continuous pain may be due to ischemia and necrosis. Abdominal distension is present and tinkling peristalsis are heard. X-rays demonstrate large dilated loops of large bowel with absence of rectal gas (Fig. 12.2). Colonoscopy and sigmoidoscopy are diagnostic and therapeautic at times as is barium enema. Caution as perforation may result. The causes include malignancy, volvulus, diverticulosis, inflammatory

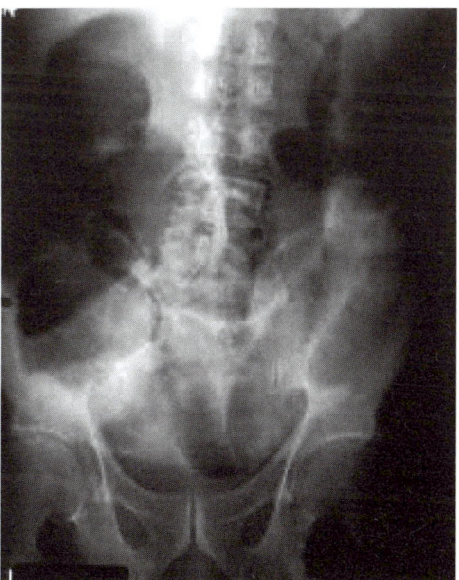

FIGURE 12.2: Large bowel obstruction on abdominal X-ray

bowel disease, impaction, strictures, and adhesions. If left untreated, ischemia, infarction, perforation, and septic shock may result. Differentiate from small bowel obstruction, inflammatory bowel disease, ileus and pseudo-obstruction.

Management

Large bowel obstruction is an emergency. Fluid replacement along with electrolyte imbalance correction is essential. Barium enema, colonoscopy and sigmoidoscopy may be diagnostic as well as therapeautic. If obstruction present, endoscopic or surgical intervention may be required. Many cases will need broad-spectrum antibiotics. If nausea and vomiting is present, nasogastric tube will be needed for decompression. In the absence of perforation, conservative management may be tried initially.

Paralytic Ileus

Diagnosis and Presentation

Paralytic ileus is absence of peristaltic activity in the gut in the absence of mechanical obstruction. This presents like intestinal obstruction with pain, vomiting and obstipation. There may be massive abdominal distension and decreased or absent bowel sounds. Amylase may be elevated and X-rays demonstrate gas filled loops with air-fluid levels (Fig. 12.3). Barium swallow is useful in differentiating this from obstruction. It can be precipitated by any severe infection, recent surgery, rupture/perforation, peritonitis, medications, ischemia, trauma, uremia, hypokalemia and acidosis.

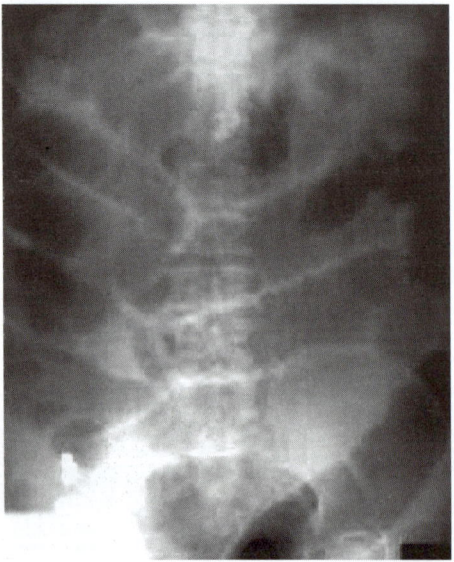

FIGURE 12.3: Abdominal X-ray in paralytic ileus

Management

If possible enteral feeding is recommended as this may restore the normal motility. Correction of the underlying cause is essential as is the correction of fluid and electrolyte imbalance. Stop or reduce medications worsening ileus. NG tube may be used to reduce symptoms. Prokinetics like erythromycin and metoclopramide may be used once ileus is diagnosed. Neostigmine may also be tried. Colonoscopy is needed if colon dilated. Opioids should be reduced or avoided to reduce ileus. If enteral feeding fails, parenteral nutrition may be needed depending on the cause.

Upper Gastrointestinal Bleeding

Diagnosis and Presentation

Upper gastrointestinal (GI) bleed is bleeding in the upper part of GI tract commonly from the stomach, esophagus or duodenum. If vomited out, its called hematemesis while blood in the stool presents in altered form called melena. Rarely fresh blood per rectum can be seen too when the bleeding is rapid and in large amounts. It may be asymptomatic but in extreme cases may lead to collapse and hypotension if blood loss is massive. Stigmata of liver disease may be present and symptoms depend on the amount of blood loss and physiological reserve. Vital signs including heart rate and blood pressure should be monitored closely for signs of blood loss and shock. Laboratory results may be normal in acute blood loss, but in chronic disease iron deficiency anemia is present. Blood urea nitrogen may go up due to prerenal azotemia and increased urea production by GI bacteria. Occult blood will be positive in more chronic cases. OGD will reveal the site and possible cause of bleeding; angiography may be needed for localization if OGD is inconclusive. Scoring system has been used with success to determine aggressive versus conservative management. If the score is zero, patients can be managed in outpatient setting.

1. Hemoglobin level >12.9 g/dL (men) or >11.9 g/dL (women)
2. Systolic blood pressure >109 mm Hg
3. Pulse <100/minute
4. Blood urea nitrogen level <18.2 mg/dL
5. No melena or syncope
6. No past or present liver disease or heart failure.

Higher mortality if old age, shock, malignancy, liver disease and active bleeding. Differentiate from peptic ulcer, erosions, varices, malignancy, esophagitis, etc.

Management

Airway and breathing must be stabilized first. Maintain the blood pressure with fluids and blood products. Hemoglobin and coagulation should be corrected. OGD is both diagnostic and therapeautic in many instances with the use of adrenaline, bands or rarely sclerotherapy. Proton pump inhibitors are needed to reduce acid production. Octreotide or terlipressin are used to reduce portal pressures in variceal bleed. Surgery is rarely needed for intractable bleeding.

Lower Gastrointestinal Bleed

Diagnosis

Bleeding below the ligament of Treitz may cause bleeding per rectum or hematochezia. The symptoms depend on the acuteness of blood loss and physiological reserve. Occasionally may present with hematemesis though very rarely. Most bleeds are from the colon, while a small proportion is either upper GI bleed or from the small intestine. Bloods will be normal in acute loss, but iron deficiency anemia is seen in chronic blood loss. Laboratory studies may demonstrate anemia. Coagulopathy should be ruled out. Drugs like NSAIDs and anticoagulants like warfarin should be stopped and their effects reversed if possible. Colonoscopy or flexible sigmoidoscopy are again diagnostic and therapeautic in many instances. Angiography or nuclear scan may be needed and most bleeding stop spontaneously. Differentiate from upper GI blood loss, hemorrhoids, inflammatory disease, malignancy and AV malformations.

Management

Most lower GI bleeds stop spontaneously. Stabilize the patient with fluids and electrolyte balance. Blood products may be needed. Exclude upper GI bleeding causes and colonoscopy will be needed if blood loss continues. Embolization may be needed in intractable bleeding and surgery in some cases.

Gastritis

Diagnosis and Presentation

Gastritis is the inflammation of the stomach mucosa. This may be asymptomatic or may present with nausea and vomiting, bloating, loss of appetite, epigastric tenderness, mild anemia, fecal occult blood and rarely malena. Causes include drugs like steroids, aspirin, NSAIDs, alcohol consumption, stress and trauma, head injury, presence of infection with *H. pylori*, reflux and pernicious anemia amongst others. OGD may demonstrate erosions and erythema. This may result commonly in ICU patients due to ischemia, stress, drugs, *H. pylori* infection and prolonged ICU stay. ECG should be done if there is any concern for angina. Differentiate from peptic ulcer disease, esophagitis and malignancy.

Management

Similar to upper GI bleeding, though less hemodynamic compromise with gastritis. Antacids are tried first for mild disease. H2 blockers or proton-pump inhibitors may be needed to suppress acid production. Underlying cause is treated and drugs causing gastritis are avoided. OGD may be required for diagnosis and biopsy. *H. pylori* infection should be treated if present. Generally, a combination of two antibiotics with a proton-pump inhibitor is preferred for this. Surgery is rarely indicated. In prolonged ICU stay, consideration should be given on a daily basis for antacid prophylaxis.

Peptic Ulcer Disease

Diagnosis

Stomach or duodenal ulceration primarily because of increased gastric acid and pepsin leads to peptic ulcer disease. There is a distinct breach in the mucosal lining distinguishing it from gastritis. This may have similar presentation to gastritis with epigastric tenderness, fullness, early satiety and may be present in gastric or duodenal area. Duodenal ulcer pain is relieved by food while gastric ulcers may not be relieved by food. Vomiting and back pain may be present. Bleeding may be severe and may present with upper GI blood loss. OGD is diagnostic. Duodenal ulcers are more common and benign compared to gastric ulcers that may occasionally be linked to malignant tumors. Higher rate in prolonged illness, stress, burns, elderly patients and presence of *H. pylori* infection. Urease breath test is used for diagnosis. This may be complicated with stricture, perforation, gastric outlet obstruction and erosion. Differentiate from gastritis, varices and esophagitis.

Management

Stabilize the patient and fluids and blood products may be required depending on blood loss. Generally the duodenal ulcers are linked with *H. pylori* infection and respond well to treatment. 2 antibiotics with a proton pump inhibitor is used if *H. pylori* infection is the cause of the ulcers. In the absence of *H. pylori* infection, OGD with biopsies are done to rule out cancer. Occasionally multiple ulcers are also seen with Zollinger-Ellison syndrome and PPIs are the drugs of choice. Avoidance of drugs like aspirin, NSAIDs and steroids is essential. OGD may also be required in intractable bleeding with adrenaline injection if source of bleeding is isolated. Occasionally surgery may be required if conservative management fails.

Variceal Bleeding

Diagnosis and Presentation

Varices are dilated collateral veins around the gastroesophageal junction, which are present due to increased portal venous pressure. History of chronic liver disease may be present and leads to sudden painless hematemesis. Malena may be present in large volume blood loss and may lead to hypotension. Chronic liver disease features like ascites, jaundice, palmer erythema, splenomegaly and encephalopathy may also be present. Anemia, hyperbilirubinemia, low albumin, increased aspartate aminotransferase (AST), alkaline phosphatase (ALP) and alanine transaminase (ALT) with coagulation abnormalities are seen in patients with chronic liver disease asociated with varices. NG tube insertion should be done with caution. OGD is required in most cases for diagnosis if first presentation. Differentiate from other upper GI bleeding causes.

Management

Bleeding can be sudden and massive leading to shock. Airway and breathing control is required, followed by fluid administration along with blood products. Terlipressin and octreotide are needed to reduce portal pressure and reduce bleeding. Proton pump inhibitors are usually started and OGD is needed for diagnosis and treatment. Band ligation or sclerotherapy is done through OGD; band ligation now preferred to sclerotherapy. In uncontrollable bleeding, balloon tamponade may be needed with Sengstaken-Blakemore tube. Surgical intervention may be needed in extreme cases and transjugular intrahepatic portosystemic shunt may also be of value in selected cases. Antibiotics are often given empirically to prevent or treat spontaneous bacterial peritonitis. For prevention, beta blockers like propranolol are used to reduce the portal pressure.

Pancreatitis

Diagnosis

Pancreatitis is the inflammation of the pancreas due to a variety of reasons. It can be acute or chronic and often has an insidious onset with abdominal pain radiating to the back. This may be associated with nausea, vomiting, loss of appetite, and later leading to systemic inflammatory response syndrome (SIRS). Tenderness and distension are also present in most cases along with Cullen's and Grey Turner signs (ecchymosis around flank and umbilicus) in hemorrhagic pancreatitis. Lipase and amylase are elevated with raised white cell count (WCC). X-rays may demonstrate sentinel loop, but ultrasound and CT scan is needed for diagnosis. Most common causes for pancreatitis are alcohol, gallstones, tumor, infections, trauma, medications like steroids and HIV drugs, high triglycerides, high calcium and cancers amongst others. Infectious causes include viruses like *Coxsackievirus*, hepatitis B, HSV, mumps and *Cytomegalovirus*, bacteria like legionella, *Salmonella* and *Mycoplasma*, aspergillosis and ascariasis. Complications include hemorrhage, necrosis, psudocyst, abscess and ARDS. This should be differentiated from peritonitis, peptic ulcer, myocardial infarction and cholecystitis.

Management

Fluid resuscitation is required and rarely may require central venous access. NG tube is needed if ileus present. Pain control with opioids is often necessary and antiemetics may be required. Nutritional support with enteral feeding is recommended early. Occasionally patients will need post pyloric feeds failing which total parenteral nutrition may be required. Broad-spectrum antibiotics should only be started in complicated pancreatitis. Pseudocysts and fluid collections may be drained percutaneously and is preferred now. Surgical intervention is occasionally required in necrosis and abscess formation. SIRS may also require inotropic/vasopressor support. Occasionally the respiratory failure associated is bad enough to require mechanical ventilation in severe cases. Early pain control, nutrition and chest physiotherapy may avoid this. Many scoring systems have been developed for prognostication. One of the simple one is BISAP score:
1. Blood urea nitrogen >25 mg/dL
2. Impaired mental status
3. SIRS
4. Age >60 years
5. Pleural effusion.

Acute Hepatic Failure

Diagnosis

This is a rapidly progressive liver impairment and generally presents with encephalopathy, sleep problems, confusion and coma. The presentation occurs when 80–90% of liver cells are damaged. It is defined as hyperacute if it occurs within 1 week, acute between 8–28 days and subacute if its between 4–12 weeks. Shock, tachycardia and fever may be present with jaundice, abdominal pain and liver enlargement. Cerebral edema with encephalopathy, coagulopathy, renal failure, SIRS, metabolic abnormalities and later shock may be present. Neurological and cardiovascular compromise occurs in advanced disease. Causes include hepatitis, paracetamol overdose, drug reaction, pregnancy, Reye's syndrome amongst others. Rapid elevation in liver enzymes is seen with bilirubin, aspartate aminotransferase (AST), alanine transaminase (ALT) raised with low glucose and albumin. Poor prognosis if very young or old, coma, multiorgan failure, associated viral hepatitis, coagulation disorders, high

biliurbin, etc. Differentiate from viral hepatitis, sepsis syndrome, pregnancy induced liver dysfunction, toxins and poisoning. King's College in London has developed a criteria for liver transplant in hepatic failure patients:
- ❑ Paracetamol overdose:
  - pH <7.3
  - PT >100 seconds
  - Serum creatinine >3.4 mg/dL
  - Grade III or IV encephalopathy.
- ❑ Other patients:
  - PT >100 seconds and 3 of the following:
    - Age <10 or >40
    - Hepatitis C/E or halothane hepatitis or idiosyncratic reaction
    - Jaundice before encephalopathy >7 days
    - PT >50 seconds
    - Bilirubin >17.6 mg/dL.

Management

Airway and breathing should be controlled and intubation may be needed in many cases sometimes due to encephalopathy. Hemodynamic stability is required with fluids, blood products and often use of vasopressors. Hypoglycemia should be avoided. Treatment of cause including antidotes for paracetamol or other drugs should be used early. Cerebral edema should be managed and often intracranial pressure monitoring is required. Head end elevation and mannitol can be used for this. N-acetylcysteine may be used in all cases, but more important in paracetamol overdose. Some cases will require urgent liver transplant depending on the etiology and advice should be sought early. Criteria as described above can be used for decisions regarding transplant.

Ascites

Diagnosis and Causes

Ascites is the collection of fluid in the peritoneal cavity due to a variety of reasons. Mild ascites can be very hard to notice; but moderate to severe ascites presents with increased abdominal girth and anorexia, fullness and nausea. Stigmata of liver disease may be present and on examination fluid thrill, dullness and bulging flanks will be seen. Ascites can be classified as:

Grade 1: Mild visible on ultrasound or CT

Grade 2: Detectable with flank fullness and shifting dullness

Grade 3: Visible directly with fluid thrill.

Ascites can be transudative and exudative. Transudative causes include cirrhosis, heart failure, renal failure, hypoproteinemia or constrictive pericarditis; whereas exudative ascites includes cancer, infection like tuberculosis, pancreatitis, nephrotic syndrome and spontaneous bacterial peritonitis amongst others.

Along with routine laboratory test like complete blood count, renal function, liver function and electrolytes, ascites fluid should be sent for examination and ascertaining cell count, albumin, gram staining and culture, cytology, glucose, and LDH. Serum-ascites albumin gradient is calculated and is low in non-portal hypertensive cases (<1.1), while high in portal hypertension (>1.1). Neutrophils will be seen in spontaneous bacterial peritonitis (>250/microlitres). Ultrasound and CT scan may be needed for diagnosis ascites as well as the cause. If blood is present in ascitic drainage, this may be due to technique error or hemoperitoneum. The causes are cirrhosis, congestive cardiac failure, portal hypertension where serum-ascites albumin gradient (SAAG) is high; and malignancy, infection, nephritic syndrome and pancreatitis where SAAG is low.

Management

Fluid and salt restriction for all cases. Diuretics are used (spironolactone preferred if tolerated) in other cases. Weight should be monitored in all cases. Paracentesis is required if resistant ascites and salt poor albumin may be needed in such cases to replace the fluid drained from ascitis. Transjugular intrahepatic portosystemic shunt is considered in intractable ascitis, while liver transplant should be considered in appropriate cases. If SBP present, treat with antibiotics and albumin infusion. Caution as any treatment may precipitate encephalopathy.

Diarrhea

Diagnosis and Causes

Increase in frequency, quantity (>200 g/day), or increased fluidity for 2 days or more is called diarrhea. Diarrhea is common in ICU settings and may have multiple causes. Infections like *Clostridium difficile* is common in ICU due to overuse of antibiotics. Change in bowel flora due to the rampant use of anitibiotics can also lead to diarrhea. Drugs like antacids, anti-inflammatories, metoclopramide are also responsible for altering the motility of the bowel. Use of artificial feeds for nutrition can cause malabsorption too. Primary disease like pancreatitis and colitis also present with diarrhea as do infections like shigellosis, *Salmonella* and *E. coli* infection. Stool examination may demonstrate white cells, parasites or ova, toxins (*C. difficile*) or blood. Flexible sigmoidoscopy may be required for diagnosis and sampling. Complications include fluid and electrolyte abnormalities, pressure sores, and subsequent infections. This can also be transmitted to other patients if proper hand hygiene is not followed. This should be differentiated from intolerances,

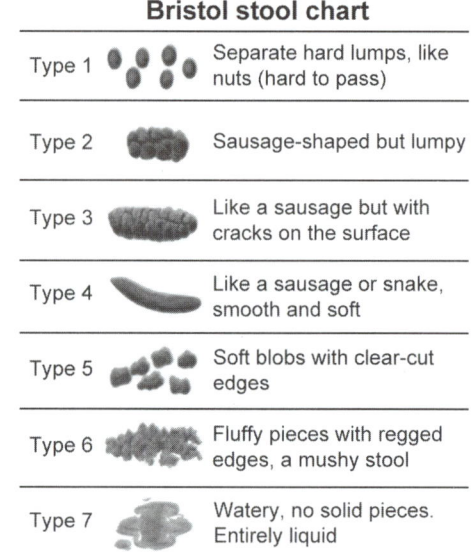

FIGURE 12.4: Bristol stool chart is used for defining the type of stools
(For color version, see Plate 1)

pseudodiarrhea (due to impaction), pancreatic insufficiency, drugs, and types of NG feeds. Bristol stool chart is used in ICUs to better define the stool type (Fig. 12.4).

Management

Correct the fluid and electrolyte abnormalities. Stop the drugs and medications that may increase diarrhea. Probiotics have been shown in studies to have some benefits with antibiotic associated diarrhea by replacing the normal flora. Antidiarrheal drugs may be needed once infections are cleared. Specific antibiotics can be used depending on the infections. If C difficile infection is proven, oral vancomycin or metronidazole are used. Isolation is required in these patients. If diarrhea is associated with NG feed, feeds may need to be changed to elemental feed or high fiber feed or changing the osmolality or rate. Parenteral feed is required in rare cases. Per rectal examination is needed if impaction suspected. Malabsorption can be treated depending on the reason for malabsorption. Inflammatory bowel diseases will need treatment with steroids and other agents.

Acute Cholangitis

Diagnosis and Differentials

Acute or ascending cholangitis is infection of the bile duct caused by bacteria. It is a medical emergency needing emergent treatment. This presents with Charcot's triad of fever, jaundice and abdominal pain. If septic shock and encephalopathy is present, its call Reynold's pentad. The pain is right quadrantric, and sepsis syndrome often present with increased white cell count (WCC), bilirubin, alkaline phosphatase, and amylase. Ultrasound will demonstrate stone, stricture, or duct dilatation and rarely CT scan or MRI may be needed. The sepsis syndrome is due to ascending bacterial infection mainly from gram-negative bacteria with underlying gallstones, stricture or malignancy. Differentiate from cholecystitis, liver abscess or pancreatitis.

Management

Fluid and electrolyte correction is essential. Some patients will need vasopressor support for septic shock. Antibiotics covering gram negative bacteria is started as soon as possible. Endoscopic or surgical drainage may be needed if medical management is inadequate. Sphincterotomy and stent placement can be done endoscopically. Diagnose and treat the cause of obstruction. Cholecystectomy is generally performed once medically stable to reduce the changes of gall stone formation in the future.

Suggested Reading

1. Banks PA, Freeman ML. "Practice guidelines in acute Pancreatitis". Am J Gastroenterol. 2006;101(2379-400):2379-400.
2. Boparai V, Rajagopalan J, Triadafilopoulos G. "Guide to the use of proton pump inhibitors in adult patients". Drugs. 2008;68(7):925-47.
3. British Society of Gastroenterology Endoscopy Committee. "Non-variceal upper gastrointestinal haemorrhage: guidelines". Gut. 2002;51 Suppl 4: iv1-6.
4. Diaz JJ Jr, Bokhari F, Mowery NT, Acosta JA, Block EF, Bromberg WJ, et al. Guidelines for management of small bowel obstruction. J Trauma. 2008;64(6):1651-64.
5. DuPont HL. "Acute infectious diarrhea in immunocompetent adults". The New England Journal of Medicine. 2014;370(16):1532-40.
6. Garcia-Tsao G, Sanyal AJ, Grace ND, Carey W. Practice Guidelines Committee of the American Association for the Study of Liver Diseases; Practice Parameters Committee of the American College of Gastroenterology. Prevention and management of gastroesophageal varices and variceal hemorrhage in cirrhosis. Hepatology. 2007;46(3):922-38.
7. Kahi CJ, Rex DK. Bowel obstruction and pseudo-obstruction. Gastroenterol Clin North Am. 2003;32(4):1229-47.
8. Kato, Ikuko; Abraham MY Nomura, Grant N. Stemmermann and Po-Huang Chyou. "A Prospective Study of Gastric and Duodenal Ulcer and Its Relation to Smoking, Alcohol, and Diet". American Journal of Epidemiology. 1992;135(5):521-30.
9. Livingston EH, Passaro EP. "Postoperative ileus". Dig Dis Sci. 1990;35(1):121-32.
10. O'Grady JG. "Acute liver failure". Postgraduate Medical Journal. 2005;81(953): 148-54.
11. Runyon BA. "Care of patients with ascites". N Engl J Med. 1994;330(5):337-42.
12. Strate LL, Orav EJ, Syngal S. "Early predictors of severity in acute lower intestinal tract bleeding". Archives of internal medicine. 2003;163(7):838-43.
13. Williams EJ, Green J, Beckingham I, Parks R, Martin D, Lombard M. "Guidelines on the management of common bile duct stones". Gut. 2008;57(7):1004-21.

CHAPTER 13

Poisonings

Organophosphorus Poisoning

Organophosphorus poisoning is common in India due to easy availability of herbicides and insecticides amongst farmer population. It can occur through inhalation, ingestion or dermal contact. The mechanism is through inactivation of acetylcholinesterases leading to both muscarinic and nicotinic side effects. This includes salivation, lacrimation, incontinence, nausea, vomiting, blurring of vision, miosis, sweating, fasciculations, weakness and ataxia. Central nervous system will be affected with headache, confusion, seizures, coma and death. Severe bronchospasm and respiratory muscle weakness may also be present. Diagnosis is based on clinical findings and collateral history from relatives or self. This should be differentiated from myasthenia gravis with cholinergic crisis.

Management

Further exposure to the agent causing symptoms is paramount. These poisons can be absorbed through the skin, so clothes should be removed and discarded. Charcoal can be used if ingestion is immediate within one hour. Airway and breathing should be supported while diagnosis and treatment is instituted. Atropine is used to reverse the peripheral muscarinic effects, but does not affect the nicotinic symptoms. The response to treatment is confirmed by pupillary dilatation and tachycardia. Up to 2-4 mg bolus is used every 10-15 minutes till response- large doses may be required on a cumulative basis depending on the response. Pralidoxamine reverses the nicotinic symptoms and is used in dose of 25-50 mg/kg over 5-15 minutes. This can be repeated as required every 4-6 hours. Patients experience full recovery most of the times. Psychiatric consult is sought once recovery takes place.

Paracetamol Overdose

Paracetamol overdose or toxicity results from suicidal ingestion of paracetamol or overuse. In the western world, this is the most common cause of acute liver failure and need of urgent liver transplant. It generally starts with non-specific abdominal symptoms of nausea, vomiting, bloating and malaise and leads rapidly to fulminant hepatic failure with low blood sugar, acidosis, encephalopathy and impending death without treatment. One of the metabolites, N-acetyl-p-benzoquinone imine (NAPQI) is responsible for much of the liver damage resulting from paracetamol overdose. Glutathione which is the antioxidant gets depleted leading to damage to the liver cells and resultant derangements. In alcoholics or previous liver problems, this can be exaggerated.

Diagnosis and Treatment

Paracetamol levels can be determined in the blood and Rumack-Matthew nomogram is used for treatment after judging the risk of toxicity (Fig. 13.1). Liver function tests are repeated at regular intervals to gauge the damage and response to treatment. Aspartate aminotransferase (AST), alanine transaminase (ALT), bilirubin and PT along with blood sugars are determined for this. If AST or ALT are more than 1000 IU/L, hepatic toxicity can be diagnoses and treatment started. Dose of <125 mg/kg rarely produces symptoms, 125–250 mg/kg causes toxicity but more than that can be fatal.

If the ingestion is recent, gastric lavage or activated charcoal can be used to reduce absorption up to 2 hours from ingestion. Oral N-acetylcysteine is the antidote of choice for this as this replenishes the dwindling stores of glutathione. This is given orally in the dose of 140 mg/kg initial dose and 70 mg/kg every 4 hours for 3 days. Other agents like cysteamine or methionine have also been used. IV acetylcysteine can also be used instead. In patients who have presented late or have already developed fulminant hepatic

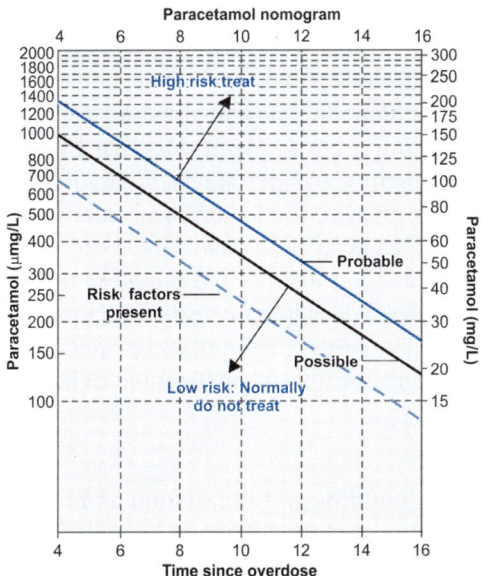

FIGURE 13.1: Rumack-Matthew nomogram

failure, liver transplant can be offered. This is decided by the actual clinical status and presence of acidosis, encephalopathy, PT >100 seconds and renal impairment.

Salicylate Overdose

Salicylate overdose occurs when large amount of salicylic acid including aspirin is ingested for suicide or inadvertently. There is a combination of respiratory alkalosis due to direct central nervous system (CNS) stimulation and metabolic acidosis due to the presence of salicylic acid in blood.

Patients presents with nausea, vomiting, pain, hematemesis, tinnitus, confusion, seizures and coma. There may be acute respiratory distress syndrome (ARDS) like picture with hypoglycemia and hyperthermia. The blood levels will be elevated and peak at 4-6 hours postingestion. Nomograms can be used for treatment. Differentiate from other poisonings, sepsis, renal failure, diabetic ketoacidosis (DKA) and pneumonia.

Management

Maintenance of airway and breathing is essential on suspicion of poisoning. Activated charcoal can be used to reduce absorption if ingestion is recent. Fluid and electrolyte correction as appropriate. Urinary alkalinization for patients with salicylate levels >35 mg/dL or symptomatic. Occasional hemodialysis may be needed if very high levels or end-organ failure present.

Tricyclic Antidepressant Overdose

Tricyclic antidepressant poisoning can lead to severe morbidity and mortality if not recognized early due to its cardiac and central nervous system side effects. Patients present with anticholinergic and alpha-adrenergic blockade leading to tachycardia, dry mouth, nausea vomiting, urine retension, confusion, drowsiness and headaches. In later stages, arrhythmias, hallucinations, seizures, shock can all present due to cardiovascular collapse. Tachycardia, arrhythmias, changed PR and QT intervals and cardiac arrest can occur. There is also decreased cardiac contractility. ECG should be done on admission and repeated as required. Prolonged QRS can result from severe toxicity and should be treated on an emergent basis. Differentiate between other drug overdoses like beta-blockers, lignocaine toxicity, myocardial ischemia, and sepsis.

Management

Cardiac monitoring should be started as soon as poisoning is suspected. Gastric decontamination is started if ingestion within 1–2 hours. IV access with, urinary catheterization should be established. ICU is recommended with all significant poisonings. Alkalinization of blood reverses some cardiac abnormalities. Other antiarrythmics like magnesium and lignocaine are also used in resistant cases. If CNS hyperactivity presents, benzodiazepines can be used. Hemodialysis can be used in severe cases.

Beta-blocker Overdose

Beta-blockers are a commonly used antianginal and anti-hypertensive medication. The main effects of overdose are cardiovascular leading to bradycardia and hypotension. Central nervous system (CNS) effects can be seen in drugs penetrating the CNS (lipophilic) and can cause sedation, altered mentation, seizures and coma. Hypoglycemia can occur and resistant cardiogenic shock can ensue. Differentiate from calcium channel blocker overdose, barbiturates or antiarrythmics.

Management

Treatment is mainly supportive. For recent ingestion, charcoal can be used. Glucagon is effective if given early with a dose of 0.05 mg/kg followed by infusion. This increases cAMP in the myocardium increasing contractility, hence bypassing the beta-adrenergic messenger system. Atropine can be tried initially for bradycardia and inotropes like dopamine and adrenaline for resistant bradycardias. Occasionally pacemakers are inserted as temporary measures. Charcoal hemoperfusion can be used for drugs like atenolol or nadolol.

Calcium-channel Blocker Overdose

Overdose with calcium channel blockers especially the non-DHPs is similar to beta-blocker overdose and presents with bradycardia, hypotension and heart blocks. Similarly, central nervous system (CNS) side effects like drowsiness, seizures and coma can also be seen, though are much more rare. The DHP (dihydropyridine group) overdose will present with hypotension and tachycardia instead. Differentiate from beta-blocker toxicity, barbiturates, anti-arrhythmic and tricyclic antidepressant (TCA) overdose.

Management

Treatment is again similar with supportive care and charcoal for recent ingestion. Calcium chloride is used for cardio protection and 10 mL of 10% calcium chloride is used and repeated if necessary. Glucagon is used in 0.1 mg/kg bolus and then infusion if calcium is ineffective. In refractory cases atropine or inotropes can be used with success.

Digitalis Toxicity

Diagnosis

Most cases of digitalis toxicity present with anorexia, nausea and vomiting. Visual changes in the form of photophobia, yellow color loss, scotoma, headache, hallucinations, drowsiness and abdominal pain are often present. Cardiac arrhythmias can occur including bradycardia, atrioventricular (AV) dissociation, supraventricular and ventricular tachycardias. Increased age, hypokalemia, hypercalcemia, hypoxia, coexisting cardiac and other medical conditions often increase the risk of toxicity. Electrocardiogram (ECG) may demonstrate the above arrhythmias and a reverse stick sign on the ST segment (Fig. 13.2). Differentiate from beta-blocker and calcium channel blocker toxicity and tricyclic antidepressant (TCA) overdose.

Management

It is important to discontinue digitalis and reverse the exacerbating factors like hypokalemia. If recent ingestion, charcoal can be used; and can be repeated over prolonged period due to enterohepatic circulation. Cardiac monitoring is essential. Digoxin antibodies (digibind) is indicated for life-threatening arrhythmias. Phenytoin, magnesium or lignocaine can be used instead of digibind for ventricular arrhythmias.

Methanol Poisoning

Diagnosis

Methanol is often present and ingested along with locally fermented alcohol. It presents with headache, nausea, vomiting, abdominal pain, lethargy, seizures, coma, visual problems and occasional deaths. Similar symptoms can be found

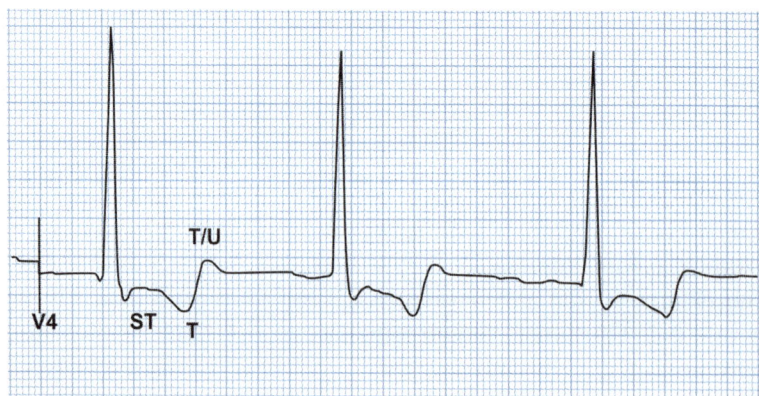

FIGURE 13.2: Reverse stick sign

in other agents like ethylene glycol and propane present in antifreeze, paints and solvents. These are all metabolized by alcohol dehydrogenase to toxic metabolites like formic acid, oxalic acid and acetone; that lead to the metabolic acidosis and cellular damage. Blindness can result from damage to the optic nerve. Small amounts ranging from 10-30 mL can be adequate to cause this damage. There is a presence of increased osmolal gap which can help with the diagnosis. Differentiate from ethanol intoxication, sepsis and other forms of high anion gap acidosis.

Management

Support with oxygen, IV fluids and full monitoring. Activated charcoal can be used if recent ingestion. If recognized early, the damage can be prevented. Bicarbonate infusion can be used in severe acidosis. Folic acid and thiamine/pyridoxine are also used in these poisonings. To saturate alcohol dehydrogenase and hence reduce toxic metabolite production, ethanol infusion can be used to reach a level of 100-150 mg/dL. Fomepizole, which inhibits the enzyme, can be used too. Dialysis is indicated in severe toxicity.

Alcohol Withdrawal

Alcohol withdrawal occurs when a patient suddenly stops drinking alcohol after a prolonged use. This can occur as quickly as 6-8 hours after last drink and worsens up to 36 hours after ingestion. The increased excitability of the CNS leads to anxiety, insomnia, sweating, facial flushing, tachycardia and high blood pressure soon followed with altered sensorium, nightmares and hallucination. Seizures can occur rarely and occasionally status epilepticus is seen if not treated appropriately. Delirium tremens occurs in about 5% patients usually 2-4 days after last drink with confusion, delusions, tremors, fever, sweating and tachycardia and may last 1-3 days, sometimes longer. Differentiate from hypoglycemia, overdose with other drugs like benzodiazepines, sepsis and thyrotoxicosis.

Management

Diagnosis is clinical and should be suspected in patients on their 2-4 days after abstinence. Acute symptoms like seizures should be treated with benzodiazepines and airway and breathing supported during the episodes. Supportive care with IV fluids is started. The mainstay of treatment is benzodiazepines in a decremental dosing. Long acting benzodiazepines like chlordiazepoxide or diazepam are used for this and slowly tapered over days to avoid withdrawal. Thiamine should be supplemented along with folic acid and other vitamins as they are usually low in alcohol dependent patients. Many patients may require a high dose of benzodiazepines. They are also used to control seizures. Delirium tremens is treated with intravenous hydration, benzodiazepines and multivitamins. Occasionally, patients may need mechanical ventilation. Clonidine has also been used in combination with benzodiazepines for additive effect. Rehabilitation is needed after the acute episode and psychiatric advise can be sought.

Benzodiazepine Withdrawal

Diagnosis

Benzodiazepine withdrawal is seen in patients who have been taking benzodiazepines for treatment or recreationally and suddenly stop the treatment. This presents with anxiety, tachycardia, tachypnea, hypertension, sweating, confusion, disorientation, tremors, fever and seizures. The symptoms are very similar to alcohol withdrawal. This can be due to reduced intake or complete abstinence or sometimes administration of flumazenil. Caution is advised in all cases when flumazenil is used as this can precipitate seizures. Short-acting agents will show withdrawal symptoms earlier while long-acting drugs may take up to a week before symptoms develop. Differentiate from alcohol withdrawal, amphetamine ingestion, sepsis, thyrotoxicosis, hypoglycaemia and other overdoses.

Management

Supportive care and IV fluids. Stabilize with long-acting benzodiazepines like chlordiazepoxide or diazepam after which slow dose reduction is carried out over weeks. For seizures again, diazepam can be used. If flumazenil is the cause of withdrawal, just supportive care is sufficient as half life of flumazenil is short.

Opioid Withdrawal

Diagnosis and Differentials

Opioid withdrawal occurs when an opioid-dependent patient suddenly stops taking opioids like morphine, heroine, codeine or other drugs and combinations. Drug dependence is present if 3 or more of the following characteristics are displayed by the patient:
1. Desire or compulsion to take the drug
2. Difficulty in controlling drug-taking behavior
3. Physiological withdrawal state when drug is stopped or reduced
4. Use of increasing dosage for same effect
5. Neglect of other activities and interests due to drug use
6. Persistence with use even with evidence of harm.

Withdrawal will present with sweating, lacrimation, yawning, restlessness, mydriasis, lack of sleep, nausea, vomiting, cramps and diarrhea. Occasionally tachycardia and hypertension is also seen. The symptoms occur in patients on regular heroine or other opioids on suddenly stopping or if naloxone is administered. Co-existing poisoning should always be considered. The onset of symptoms occurs depending on the half life of the drug in question. This can be short in cases of heroine, while prolonged in methadone. Differentiate from alcohol and benzodiazepine withdrawal.

Management

Most patients will need admission for acute withdrawal symptoms. Psychiatric help is needed for long-term rehabilitation from drug dependence. Initially, supportive care with IV fluids is started. Withdrawal symptoms are controlled with long acting opioids like methadone. An initial dose of 10 mg is usually adequate though many patients require much higher doses. Clonidine can be used as an adjunct or on its own in mild symptoms. Relapse after treatment is very common. Other drugs like naltrexone, buprenorphine and diamorphine have also been used with success in various countries.

Opioid Overdose

Diagnosis and Differentials

Opioid overdose symptoms are completely opposite to withdrawal. This occurs due to illicit drug use like heroine or overdose with prescribed opioids for pain control. Occasionally is also seen in patients who are on methadone treatment for opioid dependence who come with overdose. Depressed consciousness, decreased respirations, miosis and hypothermia may be present. Occasionally cardiac symptoms in the form of pulmonary edema, vomiting, hypoxia, acidosis and shock are also seen. Differentiate from alcohol intoxication, sedative drug overdose (benzodiazepine, ketamine, barbiturate), meningitis, sepsis, epilepsy, hypoglycemia, etc.

Management

Treatment should begin with the suspicion of opioid overdose. After airway and breathing control, supportive care with IV access is begun. Blood or urine should be sent for toxicology screening and blood gases should be done. CXR to look for aspiration and edema. If patient comatose, naloxone can be used initially to see the response. If remains comatose or signs of aspiration, intubation may be needed. Initial dose of naloxone is 2 mg in divided doses, but patients may require up to 10–20 mg in total for adequate response. Smaller doses may be adequate and regular observations are hence essential. As the drug has a short half-life, some patients may need infusions of naloxone for prolonged periods depending on the time and type of opioid ingested. In some cases activated charcoal is indicated if the drugs ingested have a long half-life and enterohepatic circulation. Caution should be exercised as this can be associated with other drug ingestion like benzodiazepines or alcohol.

Carbon Monoxide Poisoning

Diagnosis

Carbon monoxide poisoning occurs after prolonged inhalation of this toxic, but colorless and odorless gas. This gas is generated by incomplete combustion of wood and other combustive materials. The initial presentation will be with headache, nausea, dizziness, disorientation, seizures and occasionally coma leading to death. Tachycardia and hypotension can also occur with focal neurological signs. More than 100 ppm can be dangerous in humans. Cyanosis is usually absent and ECG may suggest ischemic changes. Blood gases are essential for quantifying the toxicity. This may be accidental or suicidal in which case suspect other drugs and alcohol poisoning too. As the carbon monoxide binds tightly with the hemoglobin, there is less oxygen binding and impaired oxygen delivery to the tissues. Differentiate from other drug overdoses, hypoxia, cyanide poisoning and smoke inhalation.

CO nomograms have been used to compare the levels of CO in blood with the time of exposure (Fig. 13.3).

Management

Avoid carbon monoxide exposure for long periods. Carbon monoxide sensors can be placed at workplace and home for warning. Wood combustion at fireplace can lead to increasing levels without anyone realizing. Once diagnosed, supportive care is important. High oxygen concentration is used

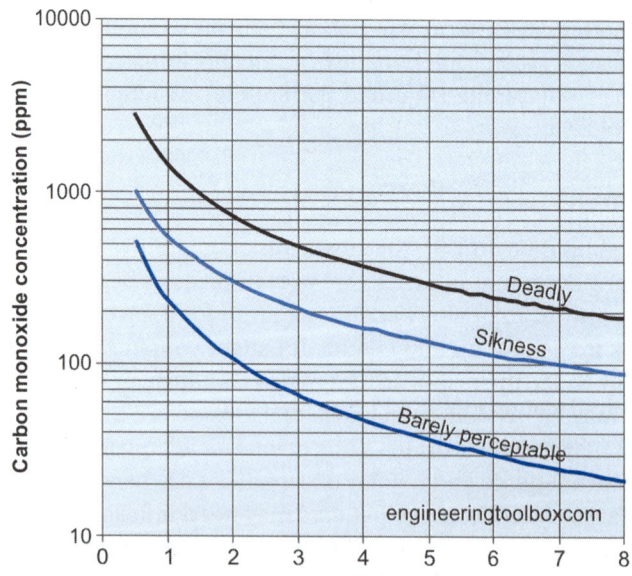

FIGURE 13.3: CO nomogram for levels and time of exposure

to displace carbon monoxide from the hemoglobin molecules. Occasionally hyperbaric oxygen needs to be used as this removes carbon monoxide even quickly, but is rarely available locally. In severe toxicity, blood transfusion or exchange transfusion may be tried. It can be associated with burns and cyanide fume poisoning too.

Snakebite

Diagnosis

Although most snakes are non-venomous, India has a few venomous snakes. Snakebite in India is common, but most bites will not lead to major problems. Most bites will occur in people working outside like farmers and fisherman. The two common types of poisonous bites are from crotalidae or pit vipers and Elapidae or cobras. Crotalidae bites lead to hematological abnormalities with local swelling, redness, paresthesia, coagulopathy, bleeding, ARDS, and collapse; while elapidae bites lead to neurological symptoms with respiratory failure and paralysis. If the symptoms are rapid in development, early treatment becomes extremely essential to save life. Differentiate from sepsis, insect bites, toxins and poisoning.

Management

If possible, identification of the snake species is important. It might not be always possible though. Protect from further injuries and bites and calm the patient. On arrival to the hospital, supportive care is started immediately. Maintain airway and breathing. Fluids are administered as appropriate. According to a national snake-bite protocol in India:
1. Reassure the patient as 70% bites are non-poisonous and 50% of the bites from poisonous snakes have inadequate quantity of poison
2. Immobilize the limb and splint it if possible.
3. Seek medical attention as soon as possible. Do not waste time in local remedies.
4. Full details of the symptoms to the medical facility to figure out the best treatment.

Antivenom serum should be procured and administered as soon as possible. Initial test dose should be given if equine serum and the dose may need to be repeated. Polyvalent antiserum is available widely in India for this. Caution should be exercised as anaphylaxis may develop to the serum. Surgical advice should be sought if bite needs cleaning and debriding. Also caution against compartment syndrome due to local swelling. Antibiotics are occasionally recommended for the infected wound.

Suggested Reading

1. Beletsky L, Rich JD, Walley AY. "Prevention of fatal opioid overdose". JAMA. 2012;308(18):1863-64.
2. Dart RC, Erdman AR, Olson KR, Christianson G, Manoguerra AS, Chyka PA, et al. American Association of Poison Control Centers. "Acetaminophen poisoning: an evidence-based consensus guideline for out-of-hospital management". Clinical toxicology (Philadelphia, Pa.) 2006;44(1):1-18.
3. De Gier N, Gorgels W, Lucassen P, Oude Voshaar R, Mulder J, Zitman F. "Discontinuation of long-term benzodiazepine use: 10-year followup". Family Practice. 2010;28(3):253-9.
4. Dugdale, David. "Digitalis toxicity". Medline Plus. Retrieved 30 October. 2014.
5. Gold B, Barish R. "Venomous snakebites. Current concepts in diagnosis, treatment, and management". Emerg Med Clin North Am. 1992;10(2):249-67.
6. Kerr G, McGuffie A, Wilkie S. "Tricyclic antidepressant overdose: a review". Emerg Med J 2001;18(4): 236-41.
7. Leibson T, Lifshitz M. "Organophosphate and carbamate poisoning: review of the current literature and summary of clinical and laboratory experience in southern israel. Isr Med Assoc J. 2008;10:767-70.
8. McKeon A, Frye MA, Delanty N. "The alcohol withdrawal syndrome." Journal of neurology, neurosurgery, and psychiatry. 2008;79(8):854-62.
9. Nicholls L, Bragaw L, Ruetsch C. "Opioid dependence treatment and guidelines". J Manag Care Pharm. 2010;16 (1 Suppl B):S14-21.
10. Omaye ST. "Metabolic modulation of carbon monoxide toxicity". Toxicology. 2002;180 (2):139-50.
11. Pearlman BL, Gambhir R. Salicylate intoxication: a clinical review. Postgrad Med. 2009;121(4):162-8.
12. Vale A. "Methanol". Medicine. 2007;35(12):633-4.

CHAPTER 14

Environmental Injuries

Heatstroke

Heatstroke results from exposure to high temperatures and causes hot skin, hypotension, tachycardia, confusion, stupor and coma. Body temperature will be higher than 40.6°C (or 105.1°F) due to problems with thermoregulation. This leads to muscle damage, shock, coagulation disorders, hemorrhages, and cerebral edema in extreme cases.

Predispositions/Causes

- Extremes of age
- Excess caffeine, stimulants, alcohol
- Hot weather
- Unattended children and adults.

Hematocrit will be raised along with potassium, creatine kinase (CK) and coagulation profile. Prevention remains important with use of sufficient fluids, light colored clothes, avoidance of direct sunlight and avoiding drinks that induce diuresis. Differentiate from sepsis, neuromalignant syndrome and malignant hyperthermia.

Management

- Airway protection and breathing should be controlled if comatose patient
- IV fluids are given appropriately
- Body temperature reduced to acceptable level with cooling methods
- Cold IV fluids and gastric lavage can be used along with bladder irrigation and hemodialysis in extreme cases
- Once the temperature is around 38°C, active cooling can be stopped
- Multi-organ dysfunction can result in such patients
- Paracetamol and other agents are not effective as the temperature regulation has failed.

Hypothermia

A core temperature below 35°C is defined as hypothermia.

This is divided into:
- Mild (32.2–35°C)
- Moderate (28–32.2°C)
- Severe (<28°C).

Mild hypothermia presents with shivering, confusion, slurring of speech, tachycardia and tachypnea. Moderate hypothermia will present with reduction in shivering, rigidity, lethargy, hallucinations, bradycardia and other arrhythmias, J wave on ECG, hypoventilation; while severe hypothermia presents with coma, shock, apnea, ventricular fibrillation, edema and stiffness.

Causes

- Environmental exposure to cold weather
- Injuries
- Poisoning
- Immobility
- Drugs and alcohol
- Extremes of age are more susceptible
- Medical conditions like hypothyroidism and hypoadrenalism.

Management

- Remove from cold environment
- Stabilize the airway if trauma suspected
- Continuous monitoring should be established and rewarming started depending upon the temperature and symptoms
- Many patients with severe hypothermia will need intubation and ventilation
- Cardiac arrest is treated as other cases and defibrillation successful mostly after the core temperature is above 28°C. Some patients will required prolonged resuscitation before successful defibrillation can be attempted
- Drugs are ineffective at a very low temperature, so in severe cases important to warm rapidly
- Hemofiltration can be used to rewarm as well as gastric and bladder lavage with warm saline
- External warming devices are also used, but may interfere with resuscitation
- Chances of developing sepsis postresuscitation are also high
- Full recovery of neurological function should be expected in all patients, and hence prolonged resuscitation is advised in most cases.

Frostbite

Frostbite occurs when the environmental temperatures reach below zero degrees celcius resulting in tissue ischemia and freezing. The superficial skin and subcutaneous area look painless, blanched, numb with woody appearance in deep areas. A line of demarcation may be seen after rewarming. Blisters, blanching, pain on rewarming, eschars, necrosis and edema occur when rewarming occurs. Differentiate from peripheral vascular disease, Reynaud's syndrome and necrotizing fasciitis.

Management

- Avoid cold environment
- Avoid rewarming if more cold exposure possible
- Wet heat is better with slow rewarming until all tissues are perfused
- Painkillers including opioids or epidural analgesia are needed often during rewarming
- Debridement or amputations may be needed but only after demarcation evident
- Moisturize the areas and use nonsteroidal anti-inflammatory drugs (NSAIDs) for injury
- Antibiotics are needed as many cases get infected.

Near-drowning

Drowning or near-drowning is the presence of respiratory failure resulting from submersion in a liquid. It can be quick and silent or preceded by distress in the form of agitation, limb movements or call for help. It can look like normal behavior in the final few minutes before drowning and is the third leading cause of accidental deaths worldwide.

This can be fresh and salt water drowning. Fresh water drowning is associated with hypervolemia, hypotonicity, intravascular hemolysis and dilution. Salt water drowning has opposite effect with hypovolemia, hypertonicity and hemoconcentration. Hypoxia, acidosis, hypothermia, arrhythmias and respiratory distress may be present in both cases. Disseminated intravascular coagulation (DIC), muscle damage, renal failure and shock can be present. Also beware of barotraumas, other bony injuries and toxins in these cases.

Management

The important consideration at scene is to bring the patient above water and let them breathe if they are able. Caution as during distress, patients may pull the rescuer into water. If the patient comes to the hospital with drowning, airway and breathing control is established first. Many cases will need intubation and ventilation. Aggressive fluid resuscitation may be needed based on initial osmolalities along with electrolyte correction. Antibiotics will be needed for many cases and otherwise supportive care in intensive care unit (ICU) suffices. Cold water immertion can protect patients from hypoxic brain injury, and many such patients survive prolonged submertion and cardiac arrest without any neurological sequele.

Electrical Injuries

Electrical injuries can be from live wire and lightening. Small currents may not even be perceived, while large currents can immobilize the patient leading to increased damage. Current passing through the heart can lead to arrhythmias and sudden death. Central narvous system (CNS) symptoms may include loss of consciousness and headache. On a local level, partial or full thickness burns can occur. The tissue damage may include the muscles leading to muscle damage, cramps and rhabdomyolysis. Lightening can result in burns in the point of entry and exit, paralysis, non-specific electrocardiogram (ECG) abnormalities, trauma, respiratory failure and death. Differentiate from direct cardiac event, thermal injuries, blunt trauma or toxins.

Management

In cases of local damage, wound debridement may be needed. Compartment syndrome can develop due to localized burns and damage to the muscle. Monitor creatine kinase (CK) for rhabdomyolysis and may require fluid resuscitation, alkalinization and possibly hemodialysis. Cardiac monitoring will be needed if arrhythmias are suspected or if there is history of loss of consciousness. Antiarrythmics are started as required and cardiac enzymes monitored. Intubation and ventilation may be needed in many cases.

Acute Inhalational Injury

Diagnosis

Acute inhalational injury is commonly present in burns patients. It should be suspected if nasal hairs are singed, have soot, face is burnt or carbonaceous deposits are present in nose and pharynx. This can lead to irritation, bronchoconstriction, wheeze, pneumonitis, chest pain, cough, and respiratory failure. There might be presence of erythema, ulcers, soot in the oropharynx and edema in larynx on examination. There can be sudden loss of airway and respiratory arrest if not recognized early. There may be increased presence of carboxyhemoglobin and cyanmethemoglobin in blood. Particles <100 microns enter the airway, <10 microns lower airway and <5 microns in terminal bronchioles and alveoli.

Lactates may be elevated in cyanide poisoning. Burns on the face, hypoxia, altered mentation and respiratory failure are bad prognostic signs. Differentiate from asthma, ARDS, pneumonia or cardiac failure.

Treatment

Airway and breathing should be controlled as soon as possible. Oxygen should be given to all patients. Any signs of respiratory compromise should be treated urgently and many patients will need intubation. Trachea and bronchi can then be cleared with bronchoscopy to reduce the irritation leading to pneumonitis. Bronchodilators and n-acetylcysteine can be used in symptomatic patients. Hyperbaric oxygen may be needed in symptomatic carbon-monoxide poisoning. Early advice from the burns unit is warranted. Antibiotics are used if signs of pneumonia.

Suggested Reading

1. Bouchama A, Knochel JP. Heat Stoke. N Engl J Med. 2002;346(25):1978-88.
2. Laosee OC, Gilchrist J, Rudd R. Drowning 2005-2009. MMWR. 2012;61(19):344-7.
3. McCauley RL, Hing DN, Robson MC, Heggers JP. Frostbite injuries: a rational approach based on the pathophysiology. J Trauma. 1983;23(2):143-7.
4. Polderman KH. Mechanisms of action, physiological effects and complications of hypothermia. Crit Care Med. 2009;37(7):S186-202.

CHAPTER 15

Skin Diseases in ICU

Measles

Diagnosis and Presentation

Measles is caused due to a viral infection from measles virus. The prevalence and incidence of this disease is going down slowly due to the immunization. This can present in both children and adults; the severity of disease is more in adults. It initially presents with respiratory symptoms and rash. The incubation period of this disease is 1-2 weeks, followed by high fevers, cough, coryzal symptoms and conjunctivitis. The skin manifestation is in the form of erythematous macules and papules on the upper part of the body and then spreads to the trunk and limbs (Fig. 15.1). Koplik's spots may be present in the mouth few days before the full symptoms develop. The initial viral infection may later on lead to secondary bacterial infections, ear infections, pneumonia, liver function derangement and low platelets. This should be differentiated from drug allergies, and other viral infections.

Management

Prevention is extremely important and has reduced the disease burden and mortality from the disease by almost 75% in the world. The management is

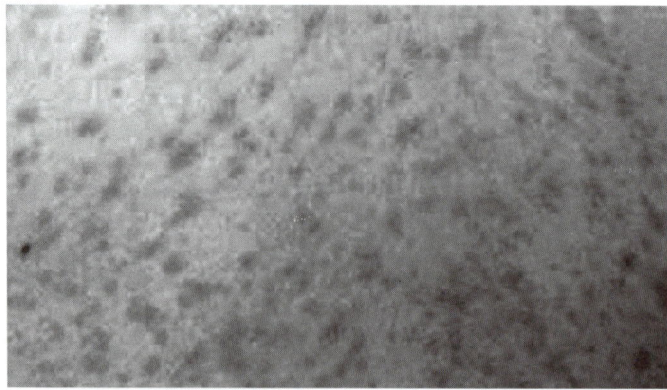

FIGURE 15.1: Measles rash *(for color version, see Plate 1)*

mainly supportive. Intravenous immunoglobulin, ribavirin, and interferon have been used for complicated measles. Barrier nursing is advised to prevent further spread of this highly contagious disease. Caution should be exercised in already immunocompromised patients.

Chicken Pox

Diagnosis and Presentation

This is caused by varicella-zoster virus. Chicken pox is the primary infection, but reactivation can also occur which leads to shingles. Chicken pox or primary varicella infection presents after 1-3 weeks incubation in the form of fever, malaise, macules appearing on the trunk and face with spread to the limbs, vesicular conversion which rupture and crust (Fig. 15.2). Ulcer formation occurs in the mucosal areas too. This disease can be severe in immunocompromised patients leading to pneumonia, myocarditis, encephalitis and disseminated intravascular coagulation (DIC). Diagnosis can be confirmed with Tzanck smear demonstrating multinucleated giant cells and immunofluorescent antibody stain. Reactivation leads to painful eruption of multiple vesicles in a dermatomal distribution. Differentiate from other viral eruptions, herpes simplex infection or eczema herpeticum.

Management

Vaccines are available and can confer immunity against chicken pox. Once the rash stats appearing, IV acyclovir is used in any complicated or immunocompromised patients. In primary varicella infection, oral acyclovir is used in the dose of 800 mg five times daily for 5-7 days. Similarly in

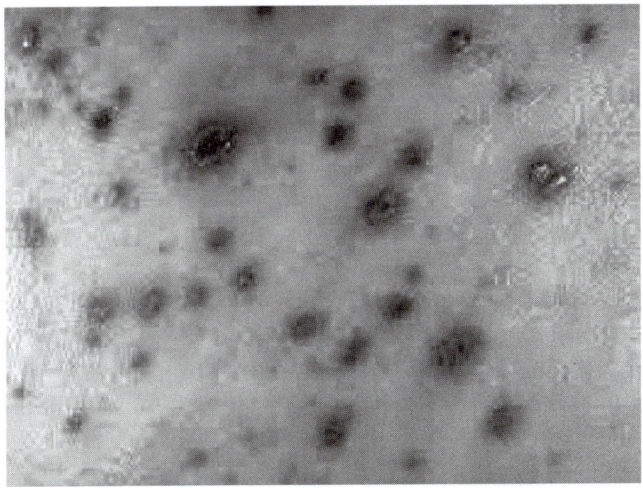

FIGURE 15.2: Chicken pox rash *(for color version, see Plate 2)*

elderly patients, on presentation for less than 3 days, acyclovir, famciclovir or valacyclovir can be given. Secondary infections should be treated and symptoms controlled.

Toxic Shock Syndrome

Diagnosis

Toxic shock syndrome is generally caused by bacterial toxins commonly from *Streptococcus pyogenes* or *Staphylococcus aureus*. This is a multisystem disorder that is characterized by fever, vomiting, diarrhea, sore throat, myalgia and shock. Skin manifestations are common and present with erythema, skin edema, skin desquamation in the soles, palms and all over the extremities over 2-3 weeks. Acute renal failure, liver dysfunction, cardiovascular instability, and refractory shock can occur rapidly in untreated patients. Women in the menstruating time tend to have severe disease and more common in people using tampons and diaphragms with staphylococcal infection the leading cause of these symptoms. Differentiate from drug reactions, measles and other viral exanthema and septic shock.

Management

Source of infection should be identified and treated urgently. Fluids are required for resuscitation along with other organ support as in septic shock. Surgical consult should be obtained in case of localized infection or abscess. Broad spectrum antibiotics are started as soon as possible till sensitivities are back, when they can be tapered.

Drug Reactions

Diagnosis and Differentials

The drug reactions generally present 5-10 days after exposure to a new drug or 1-2 days after repeat exposure to a particular drug in sensitized patients. Drug reactions are common and can occur in to 1/3rd of the patients admitted to hospital. The common symptoms are pruritus, symmetric eruptions with low grade fever and malaise. These symptoms usually resolve on discontinuation of the drug in question. Urticaria can also be seen lasting 1-2 days with pink, edematous, pruritic wheals of multiple shapes and form. Angioedema is a more severe reaction involving deeper dermal layers and mucosa. Bullous drug eruptions can also occur and include Steven-Johnson syndrome, toxic epidermal necrolysis syndrome (TENS), necrosis and fixed drug eruptions (Steven Johnson syndrome and TENS are discussed below). Differentiate from bacterial and viral infection, food allergies, insect and snake bites, vasculitis, pemphigoid, and porphyria.

Management

Identification of the drug responsible is essential, but may be difficult. Alternative drugs should be chosen. Supportive measures, fluid and electrolyte replacement along with antihistaminics and occasionally steroids may be needed. In severe reactions, adrenaline may have to be used along with fluids, antihistaminics and steroids. Topical soothing agents like calamine lotion may be needed. Future testing may be required in such patients to identify the causative agent. Serum tryptase levels can be requested to identify mast cell degranulation in severe reactions.

Steven Johnson Syndrome

Diagnosis

Steven Johnson syndrome results generally from a severe drug reaction. Erythema multiforme and Steven Johnson syndrome are in the same disease spectrum. Steven Johnson syndrome is the milder form of toxic epidermal necrolysis (TEN). Steven Johnson syndrome has <10% skin surface involvement while TEN has >30% involvement. These result from reaction to drugs and occasionally infections and present with fever, malaise, respiratory symptoms followed by symmetric eruption of erythematous macules, papules and plaques. Target lesions are present with necrotic centers, but annular, purpuric and polycyclic lesions may also be present. In Steven Johnson syndrome, headache, high fever, mucous membrane affection is common and more severe damage to the mucosa and skin is present. Differentiate from drug reactions, pemphigus, TEN, urticaria, viral infections and vasculitis.

Management

Steven Johnson syndrome can be a medical emergency. Supportive care is essential with fluid and electrolyte replacement. Fluid loss is large due to the raw skin surface. Nutrition and pain relief is needed as appropriate. Offending agents should be discontinued or treated. Monitor for secondary bacterial infections and also for development of TEN.

Toxic Epidermal Necrolysis Syndrome

Diagnosis

This is a syndrome of skin affection caused by drugs. It can be very severe and life-threatening leading to tenderness, macules and exfoliation of epidermis and mucous membranes. Affection of >30% body surface area defines toxic epidermal necrolysis syndrome (TENS) while <30% is overlap with Steven Johnson syndrome. Bullae and slough formation is common and skin appears blistered and red. The common drugs causing this are nonsteroidal anti-inflammatory drugs (NSAIDs), drugs containing sulfa moiety, anticonvulsants, allopurinol and furosemide. Subepidermal separation of skin (Nikolsky's sign) may be present. Features of Steven Johnson syndrome (stomatitis, eruptions with target lesions) may also be present. This can later be complicated by sepsis, secondary infections, renal failure, massive fluid loss like burns. Differentiate from Steven Johnson's syndrome, toxic shock syndrome, drug reactions, pemphigus and burns. Mortality can be close to 30–40% even with full treatment and support.

Management

Manage as severe burns. Aggressive fluid replacement is essential. Discontinue the offending medications, pain relief may be needed. Nutritional support is essential. Antibiotics are used after culture results. Mucous membranes and ophthalmic complications should be sorted out early with expert advice.

Disseminated Intravascular Coagulation

Diagnosis

Disseminated intravascular coagulation (DIC) occurs when there is abnormal activation of coagulation cascade leading to multiple thrombi formation and compromised perfusion of the organs. As the consumption of coagulation factors increases, there is a lack of thrombus formation which then may lead to increased bleeding from various places. The platelets are also consumed in this consumptive coagulopathy leading to thrombocytopenia. The symptoms range from bruising and oozing at the various puncture sites to large hemorrhage and necrosis. The blood results will show abnormal clotting with activation of fibrinolysis and coagulation pathways. There is excessive generation of thrombin and formation of fibrin clots. This leads to low platelets and prolonged bleeding time, clotting time, thrombin time, partial thromboplastin time, low fibrinogen and increased fibrin degradation products. Thromboelastogram may be helpful in determining the problem in DIC. The complications include hemorrhages in the gastrointestinal (GI) tract, lungs, brain and can lead to liver, pulmonary, cardiac, renal and neurological symptoms. Differentiate from thrombotic thrombocytopenic purpura (TTP), congenital abnormalities of coagulation, leukemia and severe liver disease. There will always be an underlying cause to the DIC like:

- Infections
- Cancer
- Massive trauma
- Pregnancy induced including amniotic fluid embolism
- Transfusion reactions.

Management

It is important to identify the cause for DIC and stop further insult. Stabilize with fluids and blood products depending on the symptoms. It is important to recognize whether the current state of disease is because of consumption and formation of thrombus versus lack of coagulation factors. Depending on the process, the treatment may be heparin or antiplatelets or coagulation factor infusions. Liaise with hematologists for advice and treatment early in the disease as this can lead to fatal thrombosis or hemorrhage.

Pemphigus Vulgaris

Diagnosis

This is an autoimmune disorder where immunoglobulin G (IgG) autoantibiodies are directed against intercellular substance of epidermis. This presents as blisters on the skin that are easily ruptured on noninflammed skin (Fig. 15.3). After they rupture, erosions remain. Oral lesions are also present in about the cases. Nikolsky sign is present (skin sloughing on pressure). Intraepidermal cleft above basal skin layer with separation of keratinocytes from one another (acantholysis) on skin biopsy. Intercellular IgG and complement is present throughout epithelium on direct immunofluorescence. It can be life threatening if not recognized early and treatment started. Differentiate from erythema multiforme, toxic epidermal necrolysis syndrome (TENS), Stevens Johnson (SJ) syndrome, drug eruptions and pemphigoid.

Management

Stop medications that can cause similar reactions like penicillamine. Steroids in the form of prednisolone is given in the dose of 1 mg/kg. Azathioprine may be added at a dose of 100–150 mg/day for steroid sparing effect. Rule out

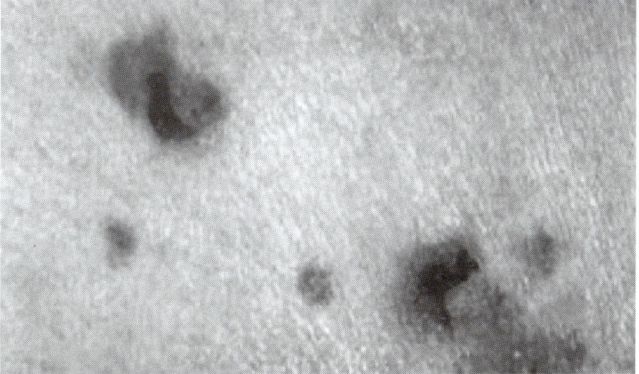

FIGURE 15.3: Pemphigus vulgaris *(for color version, see Plate 2)*

contraindications to steroids and then reduce slowly over time once disease controlled. Other antimetabolites like methotrexate, cyclophosphamide, cyclosporine, gold and mycophenolate mofetil can also be used depending upon the response. Phasmapheresis has been also used in very severe disease. Topical steroids are used in localized lesions and mucosal involvement.

Graft versus Host Disease

Diagnosis

This is a reaction of the transplanted cells or tissue against the host. This is particularly common after bone marrow transplant. Acute reaction can occur within weeks and presents with pruritic rash, erythema on palms, soles, upper trunk and then spreads to the whole body with bullae formation. Systemic manifestations are also present in the form of diarrhea, vomiting, hepatitis and malaise. Chronic reactions occur after a few months and seen as scaly plaques and desquamation, hair loss, nail changes and skin thickening. Liver function should be followed for progression and prognostication. Differentials include toxic epidermal necrolysis syndrome (TENS), Stevens Johnson (SJ) syndrome, drug reactions, systemic lupus erythematosus (SLE), viral infections and scleroderma.

Management

Correct dose and length of immunomodulating drug treatment is important. Blood transfusions are given after irradiating the products. Increased dose of immunosuppressants may be used and steroids have limited use. Ultraviolet (UV) light with psoralen (PUVA) has been also used with some success.

Candida Infection

Diagnosis

Cutaneous and mucosal candidiasis is common in intensive care patients. White curdy plaques can be seen in oral and vaginal mucosa more in patients who are diabetic and immunocompromised (Fig. 15.4). These can be painful. Angular chielitis with fissuring can also occur. Wet areas like groin, infra-mammary folds, abdominal folds and neck can also show pustules with red base and moist borders causing pruritus, irritation and burning. The chances in intensive care unit (ICU) patients is high because of widespread use of antibiotics and immunocompromise. Budding yeasts are seen under microscopy with potassium hydroxide. Differentials include bacterial infections, coating and eruptions.

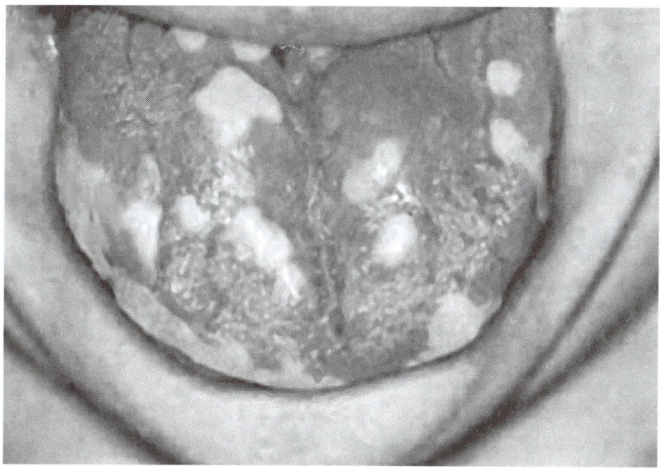

FIGURE 15.4: Oral condidiasis *(for color version, see Plate 3)*

Management

Keep infected areas clean and dry. Topical agents are usually enough to treat the localized infections. Clotrimazole cream should be used and steroid cream may be used to reduce inflammation with caution. Systemic treatment is recommended if yeast is isolated in the blood cultures.

Meningococcal Infection

Differential Diagnosis

Meningococcemia is caused by *Neisseria meningitidis* bacteria, which is a diplococci. It is commonly seen in children with an incubation period of 2 days to 2 weeks. Rash can be seen on the trunk and lower extremities and is urticarial in nature or sometimes morbilliform (Fig. 15.5). Palms, soles and mucosa may be affected too. The rash doesn't blanch on pressure (glass test). Occasionally the rash is extensive with bullae formation and necrosis. The patient presents with fever, meningeal signs, painful joints, adrenal infarct, shock, and myocarditis. Blood or cerebrospinal fluid (CSF) may demonstrate gram positive diplococci; failing which serological testing can also be done. Treatment should be started on suspicion. Differentiate from sepsis or meningitis by other bacteria, viral encephalitis or meningitis with skin rash or vasculitis.

Management

Vaccines are available to confer protection from meningococcemia. On suspicion, immediate antibiotics should be administered. Cultures and CSF

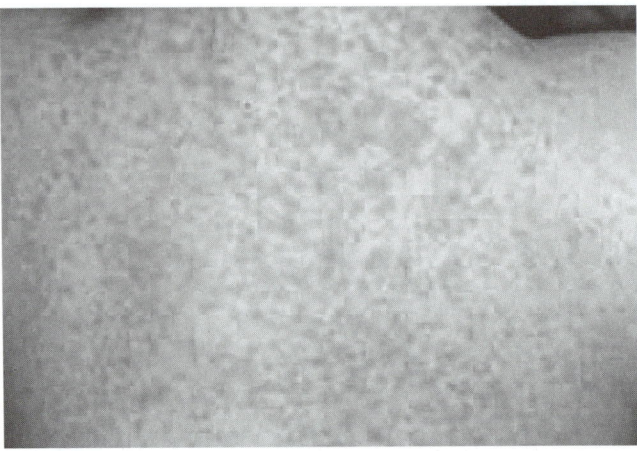

FIGURE 15.5: Meningococcal rash *(for color version, see Plate 3)*

studies should be undertaken at the earliest possible opportunity after this. Supportive care is important and may need multiple organ support and inotropes. Ceftriaxone and penicillins are used based on sensitivities locally. Barrier nursing is used and contacts traced and treated. It can lead to high mortality if not treated early.

Suggested Reading

1. Akpan A, Morgan R. "Oral candidiasis". Postgraduate Medical Journal. 2002;78 (922): 455-9.
2. Bentley, John; Sie, David. "Stevens-Johnson syndrome and toxic epidermal necrolysis". The Pharmaceutical Journal. 2014;293 (7832).
3. Bilukha OO, Rosenstein N, Rosenstein. National Center For Infectious Diseases. "Prevention and control of meningococcal disease. 230 Recommendations of the Advisory Committee on Immunization Practices (ACIP)". MMWR Recomm Rep. 2005;54(RR-7):1-21.
4. Freedberg, et al. Fitzpatrick's Dermatology in General Medicine. (6th ed). McGraw-Hill (2003).
5. Levi M. "Disseminated intravascular coagulation". Critical Care Medicine. 2007;35(9):2191-5.
6. Que Y, Moreillon Ph. *Staphylococcus aureus* (including staphylococcal toxic shock). In: Mandell GL, Bennett JE, Dolin R, eds. Principles and Practice of Infectious Diseases. 7th ed. Philadelphia, Pa: Elsevier Churchill Livingstone; 2009:chap 195.
7. Sabella C. "Measles: Not just a childhood rash". Cleveland Clinic Journal of Medicine. 2010;77(3):207-13.
8. Tunbridge AJ, Breuer J, Jeffery KJ. "Chickenpox in adults—clinical management". The Journal of Infection. 2008;57(2):95-102.

CHAPTER 16

Rheumatology

Systemic Lupus Erythematosus

This is a multisystem disease, which results from autoimmunity. Lupus is characterized by formation of antibodies to self-proteins leading to inflammation. Both genetic and environmental factors may influence the disease process. All the organs of the body can be affected by systemic lupus erythematosus (SLE). This can affect the lungs leading to hemoptysis, dyspnea, pleural effusions and consolidation. Chest pain, fever, arrhythmias, pericardial effusion, myocarditis, altered mentation, seizures, coma, renal dysfunction, joint pains, rashes, diarrhea and abdominal pain can all result from the disease. Intensive care and support may be required for respiratory, renal, cardiac or neurological involvement. Superadded infections may also result due to reduced immunity and hence early antibiotics may be required on suspicion. Many of these patients will be on steroids and this may result in increased risk of infection too.

There is no specific cause for SLE though both environmental and genetic predisposition have been suggested. Multiple genes may be responsible for the predisposition. Some drugs like procainamide, isoniazid and phenytoin can cause drug-induced lupus. Localized lupus can also be seen and is called discoid lupus.

Table 16.1: Clinical symptoms of SLE

Organ system	Symptoms
Musculoskeletal	Arthritis, arthralgia
Constitutional	Fever (absence of infection), fatigue, weight loss
Skin	Malar (butterfly) rash, alopecia, photosensitivity, purpura, Raynaud's phenomenon, urticaria, vasculitis
Gastrointestinal	Nausea vomiting, abdominal pain
Renal	Proteinuria, hematuria, nephrotic syndrome
Hematologic	Anemia, thrombocytopenia, leukopenia
Cardiac	Pericarditis, endocarditis, myocarditis
Neurologic	Seizures, psychosis, peripheral and cranial neuropathies
Pulmonary	Pulmonary hypertension, pleurisy, parenchymal disease

Diagnosis

The diagnosis depends on raised markers like antinuclear antibodies (ANA) and anti-ds-DNA. ANA may be positive in a large number of connective tissue disorders too. Anti-Smith antibody is another specific marker for SLE, while antihistone antibodies are seen in drug induced lupus. Complement levels will be low during active disease process. Other blood tests should include renal function test, liver enzymes and complete blood count. Differential diagnosis will be dependent on the organs involved as SLE can mimic many diseases.

There are specific criteria for diagnosis of SLE (any 4 of the 11):
1. Malar rash
2. Discoid rash
3. Serositis
4. Apthous oral ulcers
5. Arthritis
6. Photosensitivity
7. Blood and hematological disorders
8. Renal dysfunction
9. ANA positivity
10. Immunological testing: Anti-Smith, anti-ds DNA, APLA, etc.
11. Neurological problems like seizures or psychosis.

Management

Steroids remain the mainstay of treatment along with immunosuppressants like cyclophosphamide, azathioprine and methotrexate. Antimalarials are used for cutaneous manifestations. Plasmapheresis is used in very severe cases. IVIG can be used similarly for organ involvement or vasculitis. Avoidance of triggers like sunlight or use of sunscreens can benefit some patients. Surgical interventions like kidney transplant may be needed in some patients.

Scleroderma/Systemic Sclerosis

Diagnosis

This is another multisystem autoimmune disease with involvement of lungs, heart, gastrointestinal tract, skin and musculoskeletal system. The symptoms range from dyspnea, fatigue, hemoptysis due to affection of the lungs; right heart failure, arrhythmias, pulmonary hypertension and chest pains; esophageal involvement in the form of regurgitation, dysmotility and reflux; skin thickening, calcinosis, Reynaud's disease, telangiectasias and sclerodactyly; and arthralgia and malaise. Diffuse scleroderma is aggressive; while limited scleroderma (CREST syndrome) presents with calcinosis, Reynaud's phenomenon, esophageal dysmotility, sclerodactyly and telangiectasia. Pulmonary hypertension can be fatal and pneumonia, hemorrhages, renal affection may all lead to ICU admission. Intravenous access may be difficult. The cause of this disorder is also partly genetic and environmental with multiple genes playing a role. Differentiate from other vasculitis and autoimmune disorders, Wegener's granulomatosis or Goodpasture's syndrome.

Diagnosis is clinical with confirmation with antibodies. ANA will be positive in many patients, while antitopoisomerase antibodies like anti-scl-70 (diffuse) and anticentromere antibodies (limited) can be positive.

Management

Treatment is similar to SLE. Supportive care is essential. Steroids are used for mild disease, while immunosuppressants like cyclophosphamide is used for aggressive disease. Reynaud's phenomenon can be treated with calcium channel blockers, alpha blockers, statins, nitrates and iloprost. Malabsorption is common and dietician's advice is used. Use of total parenteral nutrition is sometimes warranted. Prokinetic agents may be used in selective cases and prevention of aspiration pneumonia with head elevation and antacids is utilized. Oxygen, pulmonary vasodilators and diuretics can be used in pulmonary hypertension. Renal involvement should be managed with blood pressure control, ACE inhibitors, and occasional use of hemodialysis.

Vasculitis

Diagnosis

The symptoms can be confusing and similar to infection, malignancy and autoimmune connective tissue disorders. Multisystem involvement is common and affects skin, mucous membranes, joints, kidneys, nerves, central nervous system and airways. Wegener's granulomatosis presents with lung and kidney affection and with non-caseating granulomas. This can lead to hemoptysis and renal failure. Goodpasture's syndrome presents with lung and renal involvement, but no granulomas are present on microscopic examination. Microscopic polyangiitis, and small-vessel vasculitis is diagnosed by presence of p-ANCA; while Wegener's granulomatosis has c-ANCA in the blood. Anemia, thrombocytopenia, leucocytosis, renal affection, casts in urine, increased erythrocyte sedimentation rate (ESR) and C-reactive protein (CRP) are all present on laboratory examination. Antinuclear antibodies (ANA), anti-neutrophil cytoplasmic antibody (ANCA) and anti-GBM are done to diagnose the specific condition; along with radiological, pathological and biopsy findings. Differentiate from collagen vascular diseases, endocarditis, paraneoplastic syndromes and sepsis.

Management

Supportive measures should be established to stabilize the patient's condition. Steroids are used initially in high doses and then reduced as appropriate.

Immunosuppression with cyclophosphamide is the mainstay of treatment if organ involvement is there. Plasmapheresis or intravenous immunoglobulin (IVIG) is used for severe disease and many patients will need renal replacement therapy. Treat infections aggressively.

Antiphospholipid Syndrome

Diagnosis

This is another autoimmune disease caused by circulating antibodies against cardiolipin or lupus anticoagulant leading to small vessel disease and occlusion. This in turn leads to multiple organ affection including but not limited to the lungs [infarcts, hemorrhages and acute respiratory distress syndrome (ARDS)], heart (infarcts, shock, valvular disease), renal disease, hypertension, abdominal pain and nervous system affection (stroke, seizures, coma). Hemolytic anemia can occur and coagulation disorders are often present. These patients are also at risk of deep vein thrombosis, pulmonary embolism and spontaneous abortions. Systemic lupus erythematosus (SLE) can be associated with this disease (secondary). Any stress like infection, trauma, surgery or pregnancy can increase the flare up. Activated partial thromboplastin time (APTT) is usually prolonged although the patient remains pro-thrombotic. Pregnant women may experience multiple abortions, intrauterine growth retardation and preterm births. Thrombocytopenia, livedo reticularis and valvular heart disease can be associated with antiphospholipid antibodies (APLA) syndrome. Differentiate from sepsis, disseminated intravascular coagulation (DIC), heparin induced thrombocytopenia, thrombotic thrombocytopenic purpura.

Management

Preventative medications include aspirain or warfarin depending on the risk and clinical state. In pregnant women with history of abortion, heparin or low molecular heparin therapy has been used with success. In acute thrombotic crisis, supportive measures should be established as soon as possible. Fluid and electrolyte management should be established. To prevent further thrombosis, heparin or other anticoagulants are used and the dose may need to be high. Ventilation, inotropic support and renal replacement therapy may all be needed in sick patients. Steroids are useful if vasculitis present or adrenal glands affected. Plasmapheresis, cyclophosphamide, IV immunoglobulins, cyclosporine, azathioprine and prostacyline may all be needed in severe disease.

Suggested Reading

1. Blotzer JW. "Systemic lupus erythematosus I: historical aspects". Md State Med J. 1983;32(6):439-41.
2. Katsumoto TR, Whitfield ML, Connolly MK. "The pathogenesis of systemic sclerosis". Annual Review of Pathology. 2011;6:509-37.
3. Rand JH. "Antiphospholipid antibody syndrome: new insights on thrombogenic mechanisms". The American journal of the medical sciences. 1998;316(2):142-51.

CHAPTER 17

Infections

Pyrexia of Unknown Origin in ICU

Diagnosis and Presentation

Central temperatures above 38.3°C is needed for diagnosis of pyrexia in intensive care unit (ICU). There may be multiple reasons for the high temperature. This includes a whole range of infections, inflammatory diseases, drugs and central nervous system disorders. It is essential to consider the diagnosis based on the presentation, clinical features and the drugs being administered in the ICU. The causes can be infections in the respiratory tract including but not limited to pneumonia, urinary tract infections, intravenous catheter related blood stream infections, colitis including clostridium difficile infection, decubitus ulcers, sinusitis (with nasogastric tubes and nasal endotracheal tubes), endocarditis, and abdominal infections. Drugs can lead to increased temperature due to drug fever, allergic reactions, neuroleptic malignant syndrome, malignant hyperpyrexia, and affect on the central nervous system. Inflammatory disorders can also lead to increased temperature as well as deep vein thrombosis. Central nervous system disorders like strokes, hemorrhages and infections can cause raised temperatures. Any tissue damage and necrosis can also cause raised temperatures including conditions like pancreatitis, trauma and burns.

Management

The treatment depends on the etiology of the pyrexia. Infections should be treated appropriately with initial broad spectrum antibiotics followed by narrow spectrum based on the sensitivities. Cultures should be send appropriately on temperature spikes. All indwelling catheters and lines should be inspected and changed is necessary. Infective endocarditis should be considered if new murmurs are present or there are stigmata of endocarditis. The suspicion should be high if structural damage present or previous infective endocarditis. Antipyretics can be used in the form of physical cooling, paracetamol and nonsteroidal anti-inflammatory drugs (NSAIDs). Cold fluids, blankets and hemodialysis can be used in severe hyperthermia once cause is established as in malignant hyperthermia or neuroleptic malignant syndrome. Infections are differentiated from inflammation and other causes of pyrexia by clinical suspicion, inflammatory markers like white cell count, neutrophilia, rise in C-reactive protein and procalcitonin.

Infection in Immunocompromized Patients

Diagnosis

Infection in immunocompromized patients are generally more severe and difficult to treat. These patients include patients on immunosuppressants, post-transplant patients, diabetics, chronic steroid use, HIV infection, neutropenic patients and splenectomy patients. Neutropenic patients have higher chances of infections with gram-negative bacilli, gram positive cocci and fungi. Post-transplant patients have high susceptibility to *Pneumocystis jiroveci (carinii)*, *Listeria monocytogenes*, *Nocardia* species, cryptococci, aspergillosis and *Cytomegalovirus* infections. Post-splenectomy patients can have infections with encapsulated bacteria like *Pneumococcus*, *Meningococcus* and *Haemophilus influenzae*; while diabetics have higher risk of cholecystitis and pyelonephritis, malignant otitis media and mucormycosis.

Management

Antibiotics should be directed at suspected organisms pending sensitivities. Clinical features should be taken into account along with local infections and sensitivities. Surgical consult should be obtained in case of abscesses and localized infections. For asplenic and HIV patients, vaccinations against *pneumococcus, Haemophilus and meningococcus* can be used with success.

Sepsis

Diagnosis

This is defined as systemic inflammatory response syndrome due to infection. Systemic inflammatony response syndrome (SIRS) is defined as presence of two or more of the following: temperature >38 or <36°C, heart rate >90 bpm, respiratory rate >20/min, white cell count (WCC) >12000/µL or <4000/µL or presence of >10% band cells. Sepsis can then progress to severe sepsis, which is sepsis with organ dysfunction or hypotension, or septic shock, which is hypotension unresponsive to fluids with hypoperfusion. Any micro-organism can cause sepsis though most often this is due to bacteria. This can be present with immunocompromise or altered immune response and is a leading cause of death in intensive care units (ICUs). Differential diagnosis includes SIRS due to inflammatory disorders like pancreatitis, burns, myocardial infarction, pulmonary emboli, malignancies, multiple trauma, etc.

Management

Sepsis survival depends on early recognition and treatment. Supportive care is started as soon as possible. IV access should be obtained and cultures sent early. Antibiotics are then administed and IV fluids started for hypotension. Urine output should be measured to check renal function and perfusion. ICU support should be sought early if vasopressor support is needed for these patients. Noradrenaline is preferred as the first vasopressor. Antibiotics are given empirically based on suspected infection and local sensitivities pending culture results. Surgical opinion should be sought for abscess and localized infections. Various other drugs are being considered for sepsis and septic shock to improve survival, but the mortality remains high.

Neutropenic Sepsis

Diagnosis and Differential

This presents in neutropenic patients (neutrophil count <500/μL) with raised temperature or other signs of sepsis. This if untreated will lead to severe sepsis, septic shock and death. The cause should be sought out early and broad spectrum antibiotics and antifungals should be started pending sensitivities. Commonly gram-negative bacilli and gram-positive cocci are the cause, but may be difficult to find in many cases. Fungal infections can also be found in some cases. Complete history, presentation and examination is essential. This should be distinguished from drug fever, malignancy and deep vein thrombosis. Indwelling catheters and lines should be inspected for signs of infection.

Management

This should be treated with broad spectrum antibiotics and antifungals as soon as possible. Cultures should be obtained if possible before starting the antibiotics including sputum, urine, and blood. Anti-pseudomonas cover with beta-lactum antibiotics, with or without aminoglycosides should be used. If gram-positive cover is needed, vancomycin or teicoplanin can be used. Antifungals are added if suspicion is high or if fever doesn't respond after few days.

Infective Endocarditis

Diagnosis

Infection in the endocardium primary involving the native valves. Lesions known as vegetations are formed with the combination of bacteria, fibrin and platelets with some inflammatory cells. This can be classified as:
1. Acute: Short incubation period followed by sepsis and septic shock.
2. Subacute: Long incubation period with prolonged course.

The common organism in acute endocarditis is *Staphylococcus bacteriae*. Subacute is commonly due to *Streptococci viridians*. New murmur, conjunctival hemorrhages, Roth spots, Osler nodes, glomerulonephritis, and Janeway lesions may be present. The classical Duke's criteria are positive blood cultures or echocardiography features plus vascular, immunological features, echocardiography features, fever and predisposing factors. Valvular abnormalities, prosthetic valves and IV drug abusers are at high risk of developing this.

The common organisms are *Staphylococcus aureus*, *Streptococcus viridians*, enterococci, *S. pneumoniae*, streptococci from other groups, *Pseudomonas*, and HACEK group (*Haemophilus*, *Actinobacillus*, *Cardiobacterium*, *Eikenella*, *Kingella*), fungi, *Legionella* and *Brucella*. Transesophageal echocardiography is the diagnostic tool of choice. Differential diagnosis includes sepsis from other sources, rheumatic disease, myxoma, thrombophlebitis and atrial myxoma.

Treatment

Once the diagnosis is established, antibiotics against the common causative organisms should be started as soon as possible. 4–6 weeks will be needed for most cases and occasionally combination therapy will be needed. Surgical opinion is sought in complicated cases with valvular disruption and abscesses, fungal infections and failed medical therapy.

Urinary Tract Infections

Diagnosis

This is infection from the urinary tract occasionally leading to sepsis and septic shock. Urinary tract infection (UTI) remains the most common hospital-acquired infection due to the prevalence of catheterization in the hospital. Women have a higher chance of this and if this presents in males, this should be investigated to find if any anatomical abnormality is present. Also seen in transplant patients, renal stones and vesicoureteral reflux. *E. coli* is the most common organism, but other gram-negative rods can be present as well as *Candida*, staphylococci and multidrug resistant organisms in intensive care unit (ICU). This can then lead to renal infections, abscess, stones, and septic shock. Differentiate from sepsis from other sources and commensals that do not need treatment.

Management

Many such bacterial growths from the urine and catheter sites do not need treatment. If symptomatic, treat with systemic antibiotics depending on local sensitivities to the common organisms. Aminoglycosides or trimethoprim is preferred, though augmentin or amoxicillin, fluoroquinolones, extended spectrum penicillin, or third generation cephalosporins are used depending upon local sensitivities. Ultrasound examination may be used to assess for abscess, stones and hydronephrosis. CT scans are rarely needed and surgical opinion is sought for structural abnormalities and collections. If urinary catheter is not needed, they should be removed as soon as possible.

Community-acquired Pneumonia

Diagnosis

Community-acquired pneumonia can be the most common reason for admission in the intensive care unit (ICU). This generally presents as acute onset fever, cough, and respiratory distress. Pleuritic chest pain may be present with hypoxia, tachypnea and chills. Chest X-ray will demonstrate patchy, local infiltrates or consolidation that may be bilateral and diffuse. Mortality is high in elderly, immunocompromized, diabetics, males and cancer patients. Presence of hypothermia, leukopenia, multilobar involvement, and resistant organisms increases the mortality. *Streptococci pneumoniae* is the most common organism involved, but *Haemophilus influenzae*, gram-negative bacteria, *Chlamydia pneumoniae*, and mycoplasma may cause it. *Legionella* can cause pneumonia with atypical features, while HIV patients can have *Pneumocystis jirovecii*. Differentiate from pulmonary edema, acute respiratory distress syndrome (ARDS), hemorrhages and lung cancer.

Management

Airway and breathing are priority. Cultures are obtained and empiric treatment started. Fluids should be administered and for community-acquired pneumonia, penicillin and macrolides will cover most pathogens. If severe infection is suspected, co-amoxiclav or tazobactam-piperacillin can be used instead. In diabetic or alcoholic patients, broader spectrum is considered as above. Third generation cephalosporins with macrolides, doxycycline or ciprofloxacin can be considered, though the chances of *Clostridium difficile* increases with the use of the above antibiotics.

Hospital-acquired Pneumonia

Diagnosis

Hospital-acquired pneumonia is pneumonia which develops after 48–72 hours of admission to the hospital. This is a common hospital-acquired infection with a high mortality. The common reason in intensive care unit (ICU) is due to aspiration of oropharyngeal secretions leading to pneumonia. Oropharynx is colonized with gram-negative bacteria, which then lead to polymicrobial infection of the lungs. It commonly results in patients who are mechanically ventilated or have poor airway reflexes. Old age, neurological impairment, chronic lung disease, supine position and presence of nasogastric tube increases the risk. Airborne infections can also occur in immunocompromised patients, so also hematogenous spread in a compromised lung. Differentiate from pulmonary edema, pulmonary emboli, acute respiratory distress syndrome (ARDS) and malignancy.

Management

This will depend on local sensitivities. Antibiotic therapy should be started as soon as possible and if possible after obtaining the sputum and blood culture samples. Quantitative endotracheal aspirates, bronchoalveolar lavage, protected brush samples are all useful and have different sensitivities and specificities. Supportive care is needed and ventilator bundles should be used to reduce the chance of nosocomial infections. Bronchoscopy, postural drainage and suctioning may be required in selected cases.

Intravenous Catheter Related Blood Stream Infections

Diagnosis

This generally presents with exit site localized infection with erythema, pus, tenderness and warmth. Tunnelled catheters may also show presence of infection that may be distant from the insertion site. The organism grown should be same in the blood culture and the catheter tip. The most common organism isolated is coagulase negative staphylococci and *Staphylococcus aureus*, but other organisms including *Candida* may also be present. Differentiate from chemical phlebitis or thrombophlebitis. This can only be reduced with careful precautions during insertion of catheter and then asepsis during use of catheter for injections and fluid administration. Remove the catheter as soon as possible from intensive care unit (ICU) patients.

Management

If signs of infection or sepsis are present, catheter should be promptly removed. The need for intravenous catheter should be reviewed on a daily basis and any such catheters that are not needed removed. Consideration should be given to insertion of peripherally inserted central venous catheters (PiCC lines) as the infection rates are much lower in such catheters and they can be left in situ for a longer period. The number of lumens should be limited to the minimum required in individual cases. In the presence of sepsis, antibiotics may be required to treat the infection even after removal of catheters.

Intra-abdominal Infections

Diagnosis

This can result from multiple causes. Presence of abscesses in peritoneal cavity, spontaneous bacterial peritonitis, secondary peritonitis, colitis, appendicitis, cholangitis and diverticulitis are a few causes of this. Symptoms may be non-specific with fever, abdominal distension, fullness, obstructive features, anorexia and reduced bowel movements. Bowel sounds may be absent and laboratory findings may show raised inflammatory markers. Computed tomography (CT) scan or ultrasound are used initially to localise the cause of the problem. Many of these infections are multibacterial involving gastrointestinal flora like enterococci, aerobic streptococci, enterobacteriaceae; while hepatic abscesses may be due to *Entamoeba histolytica* especially in India. *Candida* infections may also occur and is common in diabetics and alcoholics; while excessive use of antibiotics may increase its chance too along with multi-resistant bacilli. Spontaneous bacterial peritonitis presents with increased white cell count (WCC) in the ascitic fluid (>250 cells/cubic mm) caused mainly due to *E. coli* or other gut bacteria translocating to the peritoneum; while secondary peritonitis is more severe infection due to perforation or infarction. Differentiate from ischemic colitis, perforation, pancreatitis, peptic ulcer disease and tumors.

Management

Diagnosing the actual cause of the intra-abdominal infection is important and occasionally difficult. Once the diagnosis is made, broad spectrum antibiotics covering gut flora is needed before narrow spectrum antibiotics are used based on sensitivities. Antifungals are also used in specific patient group like alcoholics, immunosuppressed or on prolonged antibiotics. Surgical advice should be sought early as many of these conditions will need surgical input. Spontaneous bacterial peritonitis can be treated with third generation cephalosporin or tazobactam-piperacillin/co-amoxiclav; while secondary peritonitis may need broad spectrum antibiotics and surgical input.

Clostridium difficile-associated Diarrhea

Diagnosis

Indiscriminate use of antibiotics has led to increase in the rates of *Clostridium difficile* infections. The symptoms can range from asymptomatic to severe sepsis from pseudomembranous colitis, dilatation, perforation and death. Generally, a low grade fever is common with raised white cell count (WCC), and non-specific abdominal pain. This can occur in patients colonized with *Clostridium difficile* bacteria where antibiotics cause selective increase in this bacteria and lead to increased toxin production. It is common in hospitalized patients who stay for long in the hospital and are subjected to antibiotics for various infections. Two types of toxins are produced: A and B. A is enterotoxin while B is cytotoxin and both lead to various symptoms of this disease. Stool can be checked for toxins for diagnosis. Ampicillin, cephalosporins, and clindamycin are most likely to increase the chance of clostridium difficile in patients while other antibiotics like fluoroquinolones, septrin, carbapenems and metronidazole may also increase the likelihood. Differentiate from noninfectious diarrhea, ischemic colitis, inflammatory bowel disease, gastrointestinal (GI) bleed, and feed-associated diarrhea.

Management

The antibiotics incriminated in increasing this should be stopped. Oral metronidazole or oral vancomycin are the drugs of choice. Relapse may be common and may need prolonged treatment. If oral treatment not possible, intravenous metronidazole can be used. Surgical advice may be needed if toxic megacolon is present, while asymptomatic *C. difficile* carrier state should not be treated.

Bacterial Meningitis

Diagnosis

This is an infection of the central nervous system affecting the meninges. The presentation is generally with fever, headache, neck stiffness, seizures, altered mentation; but can be with severe sepsis and shock. Meningococcal infection may present with rash on the skin and mucosa. This can be diagnosed with cerebrospinal fluid (CSF) examination after a computed tomography (CT) scan has ruled out other causes and increased intracranial tension. Antibiotics are sometimes necessary before the lumbar puncture is done. The fluid might be turbid or pus like with increased white cell count (WCC) and proteins and low glucose (compare with serum). Occasionally gram-staining may reveal bacteriae in the fluid, but culture and sensitivities are required for confirmation. *Streptococcus pneumoniae, N. meningitides, Listeria* are common while tuberculosis is common in the Indian subcontinent. *Staphylococcus* is common after surgical procedures. Differential diagnosis is stroke, viral or fungal meningitis, carcinomatous meningitis or tuberculous meningitis.

Management

Supportive care is essential after the diagnosis. Hypotension is treated initially with fluids followed by inotropic support. Third generation cephalosporins are preferred as initial treatment in the form of ceftriaxone or cefotaxime. Antibiotics should be administered without delay as this can be lifesaving. Ampicillin can be added if *Listeria* suspected and vancomycin is added for penicillin resistant *Streptococcus pneumoniae*.

Encephalitis

Diagnosis

Encephalitis has similar presentation with altered sensorium, headache, fever, seizures, stupor or coma. Focal neurological signs may be present in some cases. Viral encephalitis is common with infection from herpes simplex, arbovirus and West Nile virus. This should be differentiated from central nervous system (CNS) tumors, stroke, meningitis and vasculitis.

Management

Supportive care is again essential. Diagnosis is based on computed tomography (CT) scan and CSF examination. On contrast studies, hyperemia may be visible in the temporal lobe area. Antiepileptic medications may be required in many cases. High dose acyclovir is used in suspected herpes virus infection.

Mycobacterium tuberculosis

Diagnosis and Presentation

This is caused by acid-fast bacilli of *Mycobacterium* species. Common presentation is in the form of grumbling fever, night sweats, weight loss, loss of appetite, productive cough and occasional hemoptysis. Upper lobe of the lungs are commonly affected, but chest X-ray may be normal in some cases. Reactivation tuberculosis may involve the lower lobes. Examination of the sputum may reveal acid fast bacilli, but cultures are slow to grow and may take a long time. Blood and urine may show bacilli in disseminated tuberculosis. In adults, pulmonary affection is the most common though other organs can be involved including kidneys, adrenals, gut, eyes, central nervous system, bones and lymph nodes. Biopsy is sometimes needed to diagnose the disease. The incidence is high in the subcontinent, human immnodeficiency virus (HIV) patients, poor hygiene, and institutionalized patients. Skin test may be falsely positive in many people and hence not reliable. This should be distinguished from other causes of pneumonia, Hodgkin's lymphoma, sarcoidosis, and malignancy.

Management

Isolation is required in infective cases. Respiratory failure should be managed with oxygen and if required mechanical ventilation. Isoniazide, pyrizinamide, rifampicin and ethambutol are given for the first 2 months followed by isoniazid and rifampicin for the next 4 months for respiratory tuberculosis. Other organs if affected will need longer treatment. Directly observed treatment is recommended due to poor compliance. Liver function tests and visual testing is done regularly.

Pneumocystis Jirovecii Pneumonia

Diagnosis

This commonly occurs in patients with human immunodeficiency virus (HIV) infection and presents with nonproductive cough, dyspnea, bilateral infiltrates and fever. Hypoxia is present and seems out of proportion to the X-ray features. Diagnosis is confirmed on sputum examination on Giemsa or methenamine silver stains. Immunoflouroscence can be used too. HIV infection with low CD4 counts are at high risk if not on prophylaxis for pneumocystics pneumonia (PCP). Steroids can also increase the risk. Differentiate from pulmonary embolism, congestive cardiac failure, military tuberculosis, acute respiratory distress syndrome (ARDS) and atypical pneumonia.

Management

Airway and breathing control is required in many patients and many patients will need intubation and mechanical ventilation. High dose trimethoprim sulfamethoxazole (15 mg/kg/day of trimethoprim) is needed. If this is contraindicated, atovaquone, clindamycin with primaquine, dapsone with trimethoprim or pentamidine may be needed. Steroids are also used if hypoxemia is present. Secondary prophylaxis is highly recommended in HIV patients with CD4 counts less than 200 cells/cmm along with anti-retroviral therapy.

Tetanus

Diagnosis

This is caused by the neurotoxin produced by *Clostridium tetani* bacteria. The toxin binds to the presynaptic inhibitory neurons causing uncontrolled motor neuron activity. This can be of many types: neonatal tetanus, generalized tetanus, localized tetanus and cephalic tetanus. The common presentations are locked jaw (trismus), spasms, opisthotonus, abdominal rigidity, spastic facies (risus sardonicus), hypoventilation, aspiration, autonomic disturbances and occasionally seizures. The onset may be many days after the actual infection and the risk is high in patients who have not been immunized against tetanus, unclean wounds, frostbites, and soiling of the wound. Tetanus immunization completely prevents this condition. Differential diagnosis includes strychnine poisoning, encephalitis, diphtheria, mumps, rabies and phenothiazine overdose.

Management

Tetanus immunoglobulin should be given as soon as diagnosis is made. Debride the wound and penicillin G is given in high dose to kill the bacteria (spores will be unaffected). Supportive care is needed and antispasmodic medications like diazepam are needed in high doses. Tracheostomy with mechanical ventilation may be needed if respiratory failure ensues. Seizures are treated with standard antiepileptic drugs, while autonomic disturbances may need beta-blockers. Immunization should be carried out in convalescent phase.

Botulism

Diagnosis

This infection results in a descending paralysis caused by neurotoxin secreted by *Clostridium botulinum* bacteria. Patients present with nausea vomiting, dysphagia, diplopia, dilated fixed pupils and dry mouth. Cranial nerves are affected first, followed by descending symmetrical flaccid paralysis and respiratory failure. There is no sensory dysfunction or change in sensorium and often nerves I and II are spared. Diagnosis is by confirmation of toxin in the stool, serum, gastric aspirate or suspected food. This can be food borne from ingestion of preformed toxin (onset within few hours to 1 week), wound with toxin production by *C. botulinum* (rare and seen in IV drug abusers) or in infants where the spores ingested grow in the gut and produce toxins. This toxin is highly potent and irreversibly blocks acetylcholine release at neuromuscular junctions leading to flaccid paralysis. Differentiate from myasthenia gravis, poliomyelitis, Guillain-Barré syndrome (GBS), stroke, rabies and diphtheria.

Management

Supportive care is essential with monitoring of vital capacity. Intubation and mechanical ventilation may be required. Botulinum antitoxin may be available and should be used in all suspected cases. Caution as anaphylaxis can result. Debride the wound if present and penicillin may be used in such cases.

Necrotizing Fasciitis

Diagnosis

This is a rapidly spreading infection leading to widespread necrosis of the soft tissue and fascia. This has a very high mortality if not treated surgically early. Physical findings may not be marked, but high index of suspicion is essential.

Edema, tenderness, crepitus, vesicles or bullae formation should be sought for. Patients present in severe sepsis or shock and have fever, tachycardia, tachypnea, and hypotension. White cell count (WCC) are raised, disseminated intravascular coagulation (DIC) may be present, increased creatine kinase (CK) from muscle breakdown and increased lactates. Renal failure and acidosis are present in almost all cases. This is caused by many organisms but commonly due to group A streptococci, *Clostridium* infection (gas gangrene) or may be polymicrobial (Fournier's gangrene). Diabetics, patients on steroids or immunosuppressants are at a higher risk. Differentiate from cellulitis, thrombophlebitis, compartment syndrome and soft tissue abscesses.

Management

Supportive care is established and surgical consult obtained early. Aggressive surgical treatment may save the life of the patient. Initial debridement may need to be followed after a few days with another look for re-debridement. Broad spectrum antibiotics are started pending results of sensitivities to cover both aerobes and anaerobes. The mortality still remains high.

Toxic Shock Syndrome

Diagnosis

This is a multisystem disease resulting from staphylococcal infection. Patients present with shock, high fever, vomiting, diarrhea, pharyngitis, myalgia and diffuse blanching truncal erythema followed by involvement of extremities. Skin desquamates in a few weeks including palms and soles. The infection is more likely in menstruating women using diaphragms or tampons or persons with local or post-operative staphylococcal infections. Differentiate from viral exanthema, scarlet fever, Kawasaki's disease, drug eruptions, Steven Johnson syndrome, measles or sepsis.

Management

Remove tampon, diaphragm or other source of infection. Surgical drainage or irrigation may be needed. Antibiotics are used to control the infection. Fluid resuscitation and vasopressor support may be needed along with other organ support.

Systemic Candidiasis

Diagnosis

This can result from prolonged stay in the hospital, increased use of antimicrobials in terms of length and number of agents, use of total parenteral nutrition, neutropenia, hemodialysis, external colonization with *Candida*, burns and surgeries. The patients present with fever and signs of infection not settling with antibiotics, and can further lead to opthalmitis, endocarditis, osteomyelitis and abscess formation. *Candida albicans* is the most common isolate, though other species are being isolated more and more in intensive care unit (ICU) patients. Differentiate from other non-infective or non-bacterial causes of fever.

Management

If the risk factors for fungal infection are high, antifungals can be started empirically pending blood cultures. Fluconazole is used in non-neutropenic patients. Amphotericin B is used as standard treatment in other cases. Caspofungin and other antifungals can be used in patients who are allergic or resistant cases. Indwelling catheters and lines should be removed if possible.

Suggested Reading

1. Brito V, Niederman M. "Healthcare-associated pneumonia is a heterogeneous disease, and all patients do not need the same broad spectrum antibiotic therapy as complex nosocomial pneumonia". Curr Opin Infect Dis. 2009;(22):316-25.
2. Joshi NM, Macken L, Rampton D. "Inpatient diarrhoea and Clostridium difficile infection". Clinical Medicine. 2012;12(6):583-8.
3. Kasper DL, Braunwald E, Fauci AS, Hauser S, Longo DL, Jameson JL. Harrison's Principles of Internal Medicine. McGraw-Hill. 2005;pp.731-40.
4. Mundy LM, Auwaerter PG, Oldach D, et al. "Community acquired pneumonia: impact of immune status". Am J Res Crit C Med. 1995;152 (4 Pt 1):1309-15.
5. O'Grady NP, Barie PS, Bartlett JG, et al. Guidelines for evaluation of new fever in critically ill adult patients: 2008 update from the American College of Critical Care Medicine and the Infectious Diseases Society of America. Crit Care Med. 2008; 36(4):1330-49.

CHAPTER 18

Hematological Disorders

Bleeding in ICU

Diagnosis and Causes

Bleeding that occurs spontaneously or after invasive procedures can be troublesome and result from one of many defects in coagulation or hemostasis. Normal hemostasis needs normal endothelium, coagulation factors, platelets and their function. In case of platelet disorders in number or function, ecchymosis and mucosal bleeding can occur along with bleeding during surgery and trauma. In coagulation factor problems, there is spontaneous bleeding in the joints and soft tissues. Generalized bleeding can occur in combined disorders like disseminated intravascular coagulation (DIC). Warfarin can also lead to spontaneous bleeding in soft tissue and severe bleeding in trauma. Prothrombin time is raised in vitamin K deficiency and warfarin excess or liver diseases. Activated partial thomboplastin time is raised in heparin excess, lupus anticoagulant, or inhered coagulopathy. Both prothrombin time (PT) and activated partial thromboplastin time (aPTT) may be raised in severe vitamin K deficiency, DIC, liver disease, heparin and warfarin excess. Platelet problems are discussed in separate chapter. If platelets and coagulation assays are abnormal, consider DIC where fibrin degradation products and D dimers are raised, while fibrinogen is low. Thromboelastography (TEG) can provide valuable information about the functional disorders of coagulation and guide further management (Fig. 18.1).

Management

Treatment is needed in symptomatic patients. Severity of blood loss should be estimated and blood products given accordingly. Coagulation profile should be done initially and repeated on regular basis to assess the need of individual products. Concentrated factors are available for isolated deficiencies. Vitamin K, fresh frozen plasma, cryoprecipitate, activated factor VII and platelets are all available depending on the requirements. Packed red cells may be needed in addition for replacement of blood that is lost during the bleeding. TEG guided resuscitation can save the volume of blood products administered with better effective correction of defects.

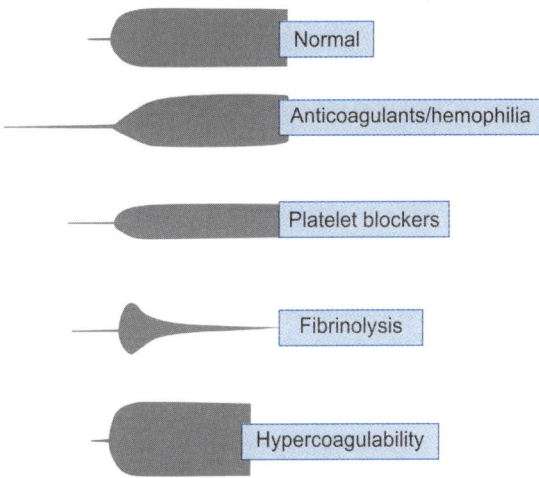

FIGURE 18.1: Thromboelastography and various disorders

Thrombocytopenia

Diagnosis and Causes

This is diagnosed by quantitative platelet count of <50,000 and presents with ecchymosis and petechiae, mucosal and intracranial hemorrhage. This can result from decreased production in the bone marrow due to drugs, infiltration with tumor or infection, alcohol, toxins and aplastic anemia; or increased consumption in severe bleeding, disseminated intravascular coagulation (DIC), drugs, hypersplenism, HELLP syndrome or heparin induced thrombocytopenia. The likelihood of spontaneous bleeding increases when the platelet count is <20,000. Differentiate from platelet clumping leading to low count, other coagulopathies, vasculitis and thrombotic thrombocytopenic purpura.

Management

If major surgery or intervention planned, transfuse platelets when count <50,000; in minor surgery keep count >30,000 and keep >10,000 otherwise to avoid spontaneous bleeding. If bleeding is present, transfuse at any count as there may be problem with the function especially if someone is on antiplatelet therapy like aspirin or clopidogrel. Caution in thrombotic thrombocytopenic purpura/hemolytic-uremic syndrome (TTP/HUS) and heparin-induced thrombocytopenia. Platelet bags are type-specific and increase the count by around 10000 per bag. Infections, sensitization and reactions can occur. In case of idiopathic thrombocytopenic purpura, steroids are helpful.

Qualitative Platelet Dysfunction

Diagnosis

This is presence of bleeding with normal platelet count >50,000 per cmm. The bleeding time may be abnormal. This can result from inherited or acquired condition. Acquired dysfunction results from use of medications like aspirin, clopidogrel, non steroidal anti-inflammatory drugs (NSAIDs), colloid solutions and conditions like uremia and liver dysfunction. Inherited causes are rare like Bernard-Soulier syndrome, Glanzmann disease or decreased factor 3 needed for adhesion. Differentiate from thrombocytopenia, coagulopathies and vitamin C deficiency.

Management

Treatment will be necessary if spontaneous bleeding present or excess bleeding during intervention or surgery. Discontinue medications and rationalize interventions. Intravenous desmopressin can improve platelet function in some cases. Renal failure can be treated with renal replacement therapy to improve function otherwise platelet transfusion may be necessary.

Heparin-induced Thrombocytopenia

Diagnosis

Heparin-induced thrombocytopenia occurs after repeated exposure to heparin. It presents as unexplained thrombosis in arteries and veins, pulmonary embolism, strokes, myocardial infarctions and reduced platelet numbers usually after a few days to 2 weeks of starting heparin therapy. Type I results in small decrease in platelet numbers in 10–20% patients and is non-immune mediated with no clinical consequence. Type II is immune mediated associated with thrombosis and occurs in 1% patients. Type II is more severe and occurs later in the course of treatment or after re-exposure resulting from heparin-platelet factor 4 complex antibody production leading to aggregation of platelets. Bleeding usually is not a problem and platelet count returns to normal after stopping heparin. Can occur with low molecular weight heparins. Differentiate from other causes of thrombocytopenia, and sepsis induced thrombocytopenia.

Management

Stop all heparins (including low molecular weight heparins) and use direct inhibitors like lepirudin or argatroban if needed. This can then be changed to warfarin once platelets are above 150,000/µL. If started early, the chances of skin necrosis from warfarin therapy are high. Future exposure to heparin should be avoided.

Hematological Disorders

Acquired Coagulopathies

Diagnosis

The presentation is similar as described with excess bleeding from puncture sites or incisions, gastrointestinal (GI) bleeds, mucosal bleeds, joints and other soft tissue affection. Prothrombin time (PT), activated partial thrombiplastin time (aPTT) or both will be prolonged. The common causes include warfarin, heparin, lover disease, vitamin K deficiency (occasionally due to use of antibiotics that suppress the vitamin K producing bacteria in the gut), disseminated intravascular coagulation (DIC), sepsis, prolonged bleeding from trauma or surgery and acquired circulating anticoagulant from transfusion. Differentiate from inherited disorders, platelet disorders, vitamin C deficiency and lupus anticoagulant (where bleeding is absent and thrombosis present).

Management

Diagnose the cause and treat it if possible. Active bleeding should be treated with factor replacement as required especially before intervention and surgery. Vitamin K is given orally or intravenously depending on the cause and rapidity of effect needed. Fresh frozen plasma will replace many of these factors, otherwise cryoprecipitate or activated factor VII is given depending on the urgency. Different types of concentrates are available depending on the deficiency.

Inherited Coagulopathy

Diagnosis

There will be a history of lifelong bleeding problems in this case, but the symptoms are similar. Family history should be explored and blood should be tested for specific factor deficiency. Von Willebrand's disease is common and is autosomal dominant with deficiency of von Willebrand's factor and qualitative platelet dysfunction and prolonged activated partial thrombiplastin time (aPTT) (relating to factor VIII deficiency). Hemophilia A is sex linked with factor VIII deficiency and hemophilia B has factor IX deficiency and is again sex linked. Other disorders are uncommon and linked to factor II, V, VII, X, XI, XIII and fibrinogen disorders. Differentiate from acquired disorders, platelet dysfunctions and lupus anticoagulant.

Management

Establish the inheritance and the cause of the problem. In active bleeding, treatment with factors that are deficient is instituted. In von Willebrand's disease, desmopressin can be used with success as it causes release of the von Willebrand's factor. Cryoprecipitate can also be used. Similarly in hemophilia

A, desmopressin or recombinant factor VIII can be used. Hemophilia B is treated with recombinant factor IX, while other disorders may need fresh frozen plasma for treatment.

Warfarin Toxicity

Diagnosis and Causes

Warfarin toxicity can result from overdose, unknowing excess dose or interaction with other drugs leading to increased plasma levels. It presents as increased prothrombin time (PT) or international normalized ratio (INR) >5 with or without signs of excess bleeding. The following pnemonic can be used for the risk factor for increased bleeding.

HAS-BLED

- **H**igh blood pressure
- **A**bnormal renal function
- **S**troke history
- **B**leeding conditions
- **L**abile INR on therapy
- **E**lderly >65
- **D**rugs and alcohol with interactions.

Differentiate from lack of vitamin K, other coagulopathies and sepsis.

Management

Treatment depends on the symptoms. If no bleeding, warfarin should be stopped and INR checked regularly till it returns to the therapeutic range when warfarin can be started again (after adjusting the dose). If minor bleeding is present, vitamin K is given orally in the dose of 1–10 mg and INR checked. If there is overt bleeding vitamin K can be given intravenously to correct the deficiency rapidly over hours. In catastrophic bleeding, prothrombin complex concentrate and vitamin K are given simultaneously. Fresh frozen plasma can be used if the complex is not available. INR levels should be monitored regularly and caution should be exercised when using vitamin K if patient needs anticoagulation due to prosthetic valves and pulmonary embolism. Oral vitamin K is preferred in small doses if risk of bleeding is low.

Red Cell Transfusion

Concepts of Transfusion

Low hemoglobin can affect oxygen delivery to the tissues. This is even more essential in patients who have end organ damage like stroke, myocardial ischemia, or renal failure. Red cell transfusion is hence necessary to increase the oxygen delivery. In acute bleeding, red cells are transfused as required depending on the blood loss and presence of other signs of shock. In chronic anemia, the hemoglobin levels should be kept above 7 g/dL if there is no organ dysfunction and 10 g/dL if end organ dysfunction is present. If the patients are going for major operative procedures, hemoglobin should be kept above 10 g/dL and blood cross-matched depending on the expected bleeding. It should be understood that blood transfusion is not without risks including incompatibility, infections and the cost associated with transfusion.

Management

Diagnose the cause of acute or chronic anemia and intervene accordingly. Active bleeding should be stopped if the source is known. In chronic cases, medications like iron, folic acid, erythropoietin and B_{12} can be used. Packed red cells can increase the hemoglobin by 0.5–1 g/dL. Watch for transfusion reactions, infections, overload and sensitization. Rapid transfusion can lead to decreased coagulation factors and platelets, which might need replacement. Also citrate can chelate calcium that is needed for active coagulation and this may need replacement. Cell salvage can be used and auto-transfusion can decrease the packed cell requirements and the side effects associated with it.

Plasma Transfusions

Concepts of Transfusion

Fresh frozen plasma is used to replace the coagulation factors in acquired or inherited deficiencies. This can be due to liver disease, vitamin K deficiency, disseminated intravascular coagulation (DIC), warfarin or heparin therapy, hemophilias, and von Willebrand's disease. Cryoprecipitate has also been used for factor VIII and fibrinogen replacement. Fresh frozen plasma (FFP) should no longer be used for fluid replacement or plasma expansion.

Management

Underlying cause should be sought and treated. If active bleeding is present, FFP can be used in adult doses (20 ml/kg) to increase the factors to 50% of normal. This means 4–6 units are needed over 4–12 hours depending on the cause. These coagulation factors will remain in circulation for up to 1 day. Volume overload can occur and chances of infection are there along with transfusion reactions. The risks associated are similar to packed red cell transfusion. Again, use of thromboelastogram may be extremely helpful in deciding what factors or components are needed.

Transfusion Reactions

Diagnosis

Transfusion reactions should be suspected in all cases of blood or plasma transfusion. Most are acute non-hemolytic reactions presenting with fever, malaise, lung infiltrates, hypoxia over 1-4 days of the transfusion or allergic reaction with rash, bronchospasm, fever, pruritus or anaphylaxis. Hemolysis can be seen in 10% of the reactions with back and joint pain, chills, hypotension, tachycardia, renal failure, shock, collapse and disseminated intravascular coagulation (DIC). This can result from incompatible blood or wrong transfusions. Chronic reactions develop over weeks due to antibodies to non-ABO group antigens and this may be subclinical and mild reaction. Other complications can occur like hypothermia, hyperkalemia, hypocalcemia, volume overload, infections, reduced platelets and immune modulation. Transfusion related acute lung injury (TRALI) results from donor antibodies reacting to host cells. These reactions should be differentiated from sepsis, allergic reactions to drugs, pulmonary edema and hemolysis.

Management

Transfusion should be stopped immediately to minimize the risk. Blood transfused should be sent back for repeat cross matching and checked for hemolysis and DIC. Hemolysis should be managed with fluids to preserve renal function. Minor reactions can be treated with anti-inflammatory drugs, anti-histamines and fluids.

Suggested Reading

1. Donahue SM, Otto CM, Thromboelastography: a tool for measuring hypercoagulability, hypocoagulability, and fibrinolysis, Journal of Veterinary Emergency and Critical Care. 2005;15(1):9-16.
2. Holbrook AM, Pereira JA, Labiris R, McDonald H, Douketis JD, Crowther M, et al. "Systematic overview of warfarin and its drug and food interactions". Arch. Intern. Med. 2005;165(10):1095-106.
3. Kelton JG, Warkentin TE. "Heparin-induced thrombocytopenia: a historical perspective". Blood 2008;112(7):2607-16.

CHAPTER 19

Special Considerations in ICU

Brain Death

Diagnosis

This is defined as irreversible cessation of cortical and brain stem function. This has to be tested by senior physicians and follow a specific rule. Oculocephalic reflex, fixed pupils, lack of motor reflexes on central and peripheral stimulation, and absence of spontaneous respiration check brainstem function. The spontaneous breathing is checked after 5-10 minutes of discontinuation of mechanical ventilation when the $paCO_2$ >55 mm Hg. Patient is given 100% oxygen to breath during this test. All the reversible causes should be excluded before declaration of brain death: hypothermia, sedative drugs, and muscle relaxants especially. These tests are repeated again after a certain time period, but the time of death is the time of first testing. Other tests can be used to determine this like electroencephalogram (EEG), magnetic resonance imaging (MRI) and transcranial Doppler; although in most countries are not required for confirmation.

Management

National and local criteria should be followed for determining brain death. Patient's family should be consulted before carrying out the test and full explanation should be provided. These patient's can be potential organ donors, so the respective teams can be involved after family's consent. Life support is then withdrawn based on the above testing. In many countries, brain death means legal death of the patient, but rules and regulations vary and local rules should be followed.

Burns and Its Management

Diagnosis

Burns are assessed in terms of depth and surface area covered. Burns can be classified as:
  1. First degree burns are superficial, red, painful and dry.

2. Second degree burns are red, wet, very painful with blistering.
3. Third degree burns are leathery involving deeper layers, dry and sometimes painless.

The area of the body involved is important to calculate the fluid losses. Each body segment in adults is given 9%, while perineum is given 1%.

The segments are head and neck, anterior and posterior chest, anterior and posterior trunk, arms, thigh, and legs including foot. Associated injuries like trauma and fractures should be sought along with burns to the airways and smoke inhalation. Specialist advise should be sought if burns involve >20% area or are in very young or old patients, involve important areas like hands, face, feet or genitalia or involve airways.

Other formulas are also used for surface area calculations (Fig. 19.1).

Management

Airway and breathing should be controlled, occasionally needing mechanical ventilation. Cause of burns and presence of soot in the nostrils point towards smoke induced airway injury and edema that may need urgent securing of airway. Excessive fluid loss occurs in such patients and fluids should be administed based on calculations. Parklands formula is commonly used:

$V = 4 \times M \times A$ mls over 24 hours; where V is the volume of fluid to be infused, M is the weight of the patient in kg, A is the burnt area.

Half of the calculated fluids is given in first 8 hours and the rest in next 16 hours. Escharotomy may be needed to improve function around the chest and limbs. Topical antimicrobials are used like silver sulfadiazine, silver nitrate and mafenide. Nutritional supplementation is needed due to increased protein loss and early enteral or parenteral nutrition is required.

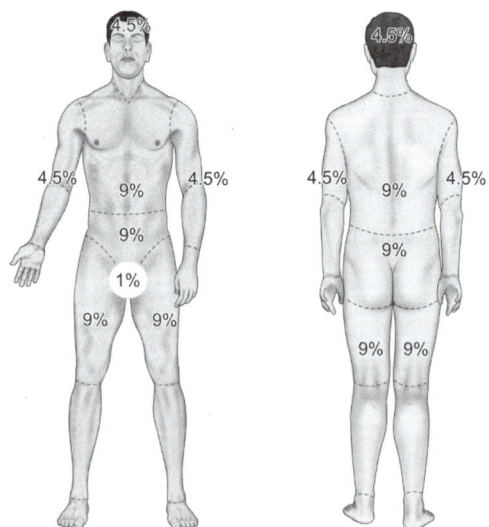

FIGURE 19.1: Calculation of area covered with burns

Patients with Chronic Renal Failure

Concepts

Chronic renal failure is defined as presence of renal impairment for >3 months period. It commonly occurs due to hypertensive disease or diabetes though other causes include glomerulonephritis, obstructive uropathy, familial polycystic disease, infections and vasculitis. Drugs like nonsteroidal anti-inflammatory drugs (NSAIDs), antibiotics, ACE-inhibitors may also lead to chronic renal failure (CRF) over time. Patients have increased urea and creatinine present over months to years. They present with malaise, nausea, hiccups, confusion, hypertension, fluid overload, pericardial effusion, asterixis, anemia, platelet dysfunction, acidosis, hyperkalemia and hypocalcemia. Ultrasound may demonstrate small kidneys, polycystic disease or obstruction.

Stages of CRF are:
- Stage 1: Reduced renal function with normal GFR >90 mL/min/1.73 m^2 BSA
- Stage 2: Mild reduction in GFR to 60–80 mL/min/1.73 m^2 BSA
- Stage 3: Moderate reduction in GFR to 30–59 mL/min/1.73 m^2 BSA
- Stage 4: Severe reduction in GFR to 15–29 mL/min/1.73 m^2 BSA
- Stage 5: ESRD or dialysis dependence or GFR <15 mL/min/1.73 m^2 BSA

Management

Fluid and electrolyte balance should be maintained. Blood pressure is controlled to reduce further damage. Sodium, protein and fluid restriction may be necessary. Hypotension should be avoided as well as nephrotoxic medications like NSAIDs, ACE-inhibitors and contrast agents. Dose may need to be adjusted for many drugs due to elimination from the kidneys. Metabolic acidosis should be controlled and may need renal replacement therapy. Other indications for hemodialysis are hyperkalemia, overload, uremic encephalopathy or other organ dysfunction. Erythropoietin is given for chronic anemia resulting from renal failure. Renal transplantation may be considered in specific cases.

Pregnant Patients in ICU

Concepts

There are many physiological changes relating to pregnancy and the presence of fetus makes management challenging. The cardiac output is raised along with total blood volume. Heart rate and stroke volume increases while the peripheral resistance is reduced. The minute volume increases leading to respiratory alkalosis, which is compensated. Dilutional anemia is present due to increased plasma volume and a prothrombotic state develops. Renal output increases leading to increased creatinine clearance while alkaline phosphatase is increased.

Management

Complete supine position should be avoided as this leads to decreased venous return. Obstetric opinion should be sought early and fetal monitoring should be established in intensive care unit (ICU). Thromboprophylaxis is essential due to increased risk and nutrition should be established for fetal growth. Radiation should be avoided if possible as this can lead to fetal defects. All the medications should be checked for teratogenicity.

Transplant Patients in ICU

Concepts

Patients who have had transplants present specific problems related to organ function, anatomical variations from the transplant and immunosuppressive therapy they are receiving. Graft failure and chronic rejection can result post-transplant; but infections remain the main concern. Initial infections are usually from bacteria, while viruses like cytomegalovirus (CMV), Epstein-Barr virus (EBV) and opportunistic infections occur in the next few months. Classic findings may not be present due to immunosuppression. Pancreatitis and hepatotoxicity may be present, while immunosuppression can also lead to malignancies like Kaposi's sarcoma and lymphoproliferative disorders. Steroids can lead to increased risk of infections, adrenal suppression, osteoporosis and diabetes. Any medications that are given in intensive care unit (ICU) should be checked for interactions with the immunosuppressive drugs. Also the vascularity to the graft should be checked with Doppler ultrasound when possible. Multidisciplinary management with transplant physicians, transplant surgeons and intensivists is essential for reduction in mortality and morbidity in these patients.

Management

All the medications that the patient is on should be continued till expert advice is sought. Any suspected infections should be treated aggressively and if this is life-threatening, immunosuppressants can be discontinued. Steroid dosage may need to be increased. Drug interactions should be carefully looked at to avoid toxicity. Biopsies are occasionally needed to check for rejection and immunosuppressive therapy may need to be increased.

Care of Elderly Patients

Concepts

Elderly patients presenting to the intensive care unit (ICU) will have co-morbid illnesses. Many of such patients will be arteriopathic and with a reduced physiological reserve. They have a reduced lung capacity and FEV1. Most patients suffer from cardiac diseases and are hypertensive. Drug metabolism is reduced and renal function is reduced. Delirium is more common in these patients more so if they have had previous strokes and are on medications. They are more prone to deep vein thrombosis (DVT), ulcers, malnutrition, falls and fractures, renal dysfunction, delirium and muscular atrophy over time. The mortality and morbidity remains high in this subset of patients.

Management

Medications should be adjusted in elderly patients in accordance with renal function, liver function and physiological reserves. The initial signs and symptoms are subtler. Home medications should be checked rigorously and started as appropriate. Opioids, sedatives and drugs affecting the nervous system should be prescribed with caution. Sleep patterns should be maintained as normal if possible to avoid delirium. Family should be involved to reduce confusion. Care should especially be taken for confusion and delirium in these patients. Also many of these patients will be at a high risk for falls and fractures and appropriate precautions should be taken to prevent these.

Obese Patients

Concepts

Obese patients are prone to have more complications and mortality in intensive care unit (ICU). Different classes of obesity are defined based on body mass index.
- BMI >25 is overweight
- BMI >30 but <35 is class I obesity
- BMI >35 but <40 is class II obesity
- BMI >40 is class III or morbid obesity.

They have a higher risk of obstructive sleep apnea, lung disease and hypoventilation syndrome. The risk for malignancy, cardiac disease, hypertension, diabetes, respiratory failure, deep vein thrombosis (DVT), pulmonary embolism (PE), ulcers and liver disorders is all increased with obesity. Intubation can be a challenge if required and also weaning from ventilation is difficult. Drug dosing may be a problem along with calculation of fluid, nutritional and electrolyte intake. Transport of these patients for investigations, procedures and scans can present itself with a challenge. Any procedure being done on these patients will be difficult and imaging may be difficult with them too. There basal metabolic rate (BMR) and oxygen demand is much higher than non-obese patients. Due to this, they will desaturate quickly and extreme caution is needed during intubation and ventilation of these patient.

Management

Drug dosage calculation may be done with ideal body weight rather than actual weight. Equipment for difficult airway and specialist help with weaning may be required. Nutritional and fluid calculations can be again estimated based on ideal weight. Special equipment may be needed with every intervention and transfer. Many of these patients will need an invasive arterial line as non-invasive blood pressure readings are difficult and inaccurate. Similarly for IV access, occasionally they will need central venous access which again can be difficult to obtain.

Suggested Reading

1. Brunicardi, Charles. "Chapter 8: Burns". Schwartz's principles of surgery (9th ed.). New York: McGraw-Hill, Medical Pub. Division (2010).
2. Qaseem A, Hopkins RH, Sweet DE, Starkey M, Shekelle P. "Screening, Monitoring, and Treatment of Stage 1 to 4 Chronic Kidney Disease: A Clinical Practice Guideline From the Clinical Guidelines Committee of the American College of Physicians". Annals of internal medicine. 2013;159(12):835-47.

CHAPTER 20

Respiratory Disorders and Management in ICU

Pneumothorax

Diagnosis

Pneumothorax results from collection of air between the pleural spaces leading to collapse of the lung due to rupture of lungs or chest wall injury. This presents with shortness of breath, pain, hypoxia, hypercarbia and air hunger. The chest will be resonant on the side of pneumothorax and breath sounds will be decreased. In tension pneumothorax, trachea will be shifted to the other side, shock and cardiac arrest may ensue due to reduced venous return. Causes include trauma, spontaneous, infections like tuberculosis, pneumocystis carinii, interventions like central line insertion, surgery, lung biopsy and mechanical ventilation. This is confirmed with a chest X-ray (Fig. 20.1), but if tension pneumothorax present immediate treatment is warranted without X-ray confirmation. Differentiate from pleural effusion, emboli or pneumonia.

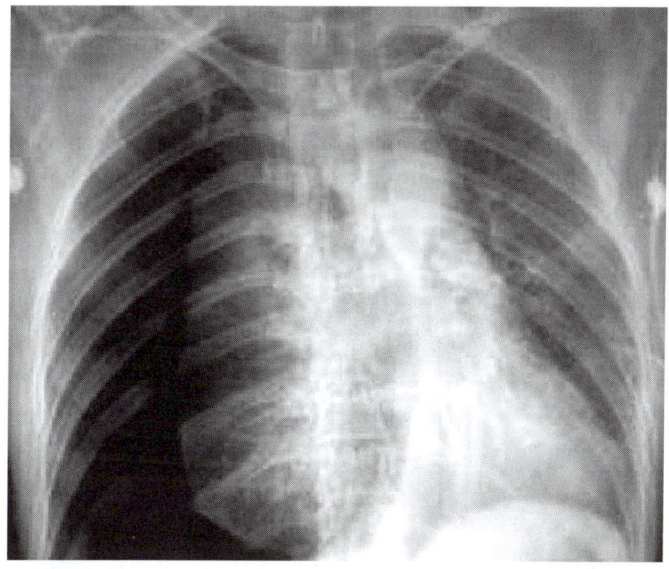

FIGURE 20.1: Pneumothorax

Management

Airway and oxygenation is important. If small pneumothorax and no accumulation, observation may be sufficient. If mechanically ventilated, intercostal drain is mostly necessary. In moderate size pneumothorax and spontaneously breathing, small size drain is sufficient. All other patients and patients on mechanical ventilation will need surgical intercostal drain. If tension pneumothorax, initial decompression can be done with a needle in the anterior chest followed by a drain.

Pleural Effusion

Diagnosis

Collection of fluid instead of air leads to pleural effusion. Symptoms depend on the rate of accumulation and are shortness of breath, pain and later respiratory failure. Chest X-ray will demonstrate presence of fluid if large collection (Fig. 20.1), but ultrasound and computed tomography (CT) scan more sensitive. X-rays in intensive care unit (ICU) are generally anteroposterior and may miss small effusions; but loss of costophrenic angle suggests accumulation of 200 mL fluid or more. Smaller effusions are seen with CT scans and ultrasound scans. Common reasons for accumulation of fluid are congestive cardiac failure, pneumonia, renal failure, tuberculosis and rarely malignancy. Generally safe to remove fluid in intensive care, but caution should be exercised in ventilated patients and small effusions. Differentiate from alelectasis, pneumonia, elevated diaphragm and thickening.

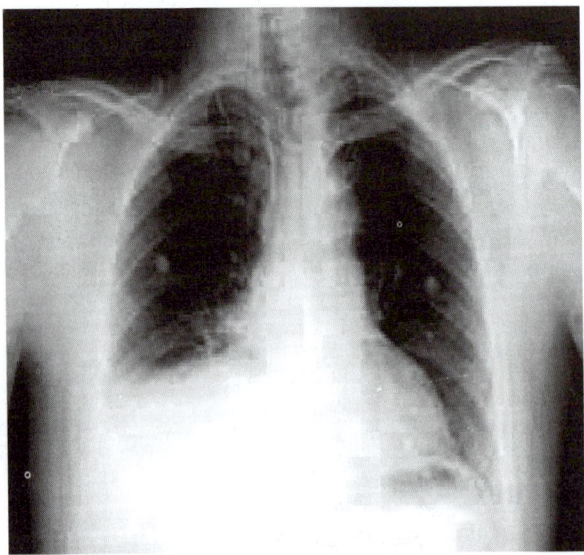

FIGURE 20.2: Pleural effusion as seen on CXR

Fluid is defined as transudate or exudate based on Light's criteria. According to this criteria, exudative effusion will have one of the following:
1. Ratio of pleural fluid protein to serum protein is greater than 0.5.
2. Ratio of pleural fluid lactate dehydrogenase (LDH) and serum LDH is greater than 0.6.
3. Pleural fluid LDH 2/3rd or more of the upper limit for serum LDH.

Management

Diagnostic pleurcentesis may be required in undiagnosed effusions. If uncomplicated, antibiotics and diuretics may be enough to resolve the effusions. If respiratory compromise present or if weaning from respiratory support difficult, may need pleural tapping even from small effusions. For larger effusions, care needs to be exercised as rapid removal of fluid may lead to pulmonary edema.

Positive End-expiratory Pressure

Concepts

The PEEP is defined as the positive end-expiratory pressure (PEEP) when mechanical ventilation is used. This is the pressure at the end of expiration in a patient. In a spontaneously breathing person, this is also called continuous positive airway pressure (CPAP). The usefulness is in reversing the atelectasis caused by various pathologies on the lung and hence increases the available area for ventilation. This thus reduces V/Q mismatch and dead space during ventilation. It also decreases the work of breathing in circumstances where the lung compliance is reduced. In cardiac failure it reduces the preload and decreases the cardiac workload, but at the same time may reduce the venous return and hence cardiac output in some situations. The Figure 20.3 demonstrates the PEEP in a normal ventilatory breath.

Uses and Management

The PEEP is normally used in all ventilated patients. If the lung function is normal, a PEEP of 5 cm is used. In obstructive disease patients, a lower PEEP may have to be used to reduce hyperinflation. In patients where oxygenation is an issue like in acute respiratory distress syndrome (ARDS) and pneumonia, higher PEEP is used to improve oxygenation and reduce FiO_2. Higher PEEP can lead to hypotension, low cardiac output, barotraumas, pneumothorax and pneumomediastinum.

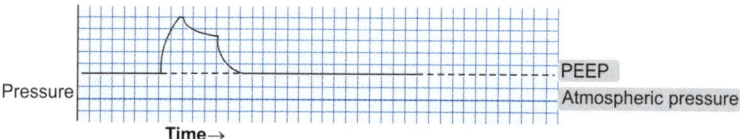

FIGURE 20.3: Pressure-time curve demonstrating PEEP during ventilatory breath

Noninvasive Ventilation

Concepts

This is delivery of positive-pressure ventilation without endotracheal tube or tracheostomy tube. This is provided via a face or nasal mask (Fig. 20.4). The successful provision of noninvasive ventilation depends on a relatively cooperative and alert patient and proper fitting of the mask. Continuous positive airway pressure delivers pressure during both inspiration and expiration. This can be provided alone and decreases the preload and work of breathing in cardiogenic pulmonary edema and other cases of respiratory failure. Inspiratory pressure can be augmented in bilevel ventilatory modes. This is more helpful in chronic airway disease patients, obstructive sleep apnea and during weaning from ventilatory support. This form of ventilation is not so useful in uncooperative patients, comatose or septic patients, excess secretions or patients with facial trauma and abnormalities. Complications include skin breakdown, aspiration, sinus infection and worsened respiratory failure.

Management

Continuous positive airway pressure (CPAP) via facemask or nasal mask is the treatment of choice in obstructive sleep apnea. It is also useful in cardiogenic pulmonary edema and restrictive lung disease. In obstructive lung disease ventilation with bilevel features is useful to reduce the respiratory acidosis. The noninvasive ventilation prevents the use of invasive devices and further complications related to endotracheal tubes and sedation.

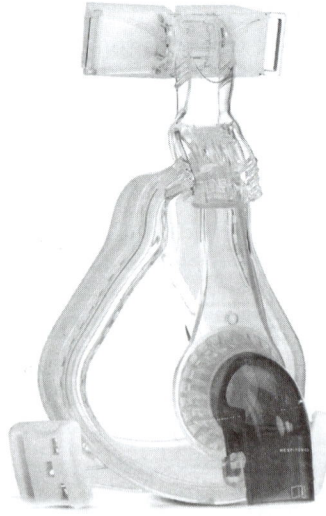

FIGURE 20.4: Noninvasive ventilation mask

Invasive Ventilation

Concepts

This is delivered with endotracheal tube or a tracheostomy tube. This is defined with the use of trigger (change from expiration to inspiration) and mode (change from inspiration to expiration). Volume-control ventilation (VCV) is the common mode with preset tidal volume every breath and preset number of breaths per minute. Patient may trigger own breaths. Pressure control ventilation (PCV) is at a set pressure and preset breaths per minute. Again patient may trigger own breath at a set pressure. Pressure support ventilation (PSV) provides a preset pressure on patients own triggered breaths. This is useful while weaning the patient from fully supported ventilation. Intermittent mandatory ventilation provides preset breaths per minute and patient can breathe spontaneously with or without support synchronized intermittent mandatory ventilation (SIMV) and again is used in weaning. There are many indications for the use of invasive ventilation including postoperative, respiratory failure, septic shock, overdose, fatigue, etc. The complications include infection, trauma, muscle weakness, neuropathy, complications related to sedation, hypotension, barotrauma and lung injury.

Management

Once the decision has been made to provide invasive mechanical ventilation, preparation is paramount before the patient is sedated and ventilated. This includes preparation for the endotracheal tube placement, use of drugs for induction and maintenance of sedation and setting the ventilator. The mode of ventilation can be chosen based on the clinical indication. Pressure control modes are used more in intensive care unit (ICU), but new modes with combination of the above modes are becoming more popular now including pressure regulated volume control (PRVC) and bilevel positive airway pressure (BiPAP).

Acute Severe Asthma

Diagnosis

Asthma not responsive or poorly responsive to therapy is acute severe asthma with severely reduced FEV1, forced vital capacity (FVC) and peak flow. This results in hypoxia and may have hypercapnia from respiratory failure and fatigue. There is very poor ventilation, with severe wheeze or silent chest, hyperinflated lungs, use of accessory muscles and pulsus paradoxus. This may be sudden worsening or a slow decline in respiratory failure. Differentiate from stridor, upper airway obstruction, vocal cord palsy, chronic obstructive pulmonary disease (COPD) and pulmonary edema.

Management

Oxygen supplementation and salbutamol nebulizers are the mainstay of treatment. This can be repeated as often as required initially and then spaced out, ipratropium is added and given in nebulized form initially. Systemic steroids like prednisolone are started but take some time to take effect. This is started at a dose of 40–60 mg. Antibiotics are only given if there are signs of infection with fever, pneumonia and purulent sputum. IV magnesium sulfate can be tried in a dose of 2–8 grams every 4–6 hours. Intravenous salbutamol has been tried in severe cases unresponsive to above treatment, but side-effects are common. Aminophylline can also be tried with caution. Patients not responding to these measures may need noninvasive or invasive ventilation. Ketamine and inhalational anesthetic drugs can also relieve the bronchospasm in some cases.

Ventilation in Acute Severe Asthma

Concepts

Ventilation is rarely required in asthmatic patients due to respiratory fatigue when the symptoms are not being relieved by medications quickly. Risk of barotrauma increases due to retention of air and hyperinflation, high pressures and leads to hypotension and acidosis. Thus the ventilation should cater to reducing the hyperinflation and reduce the work of breathing, while the drugs take effect. Hypercapnia may persist during the ventilation and should be accepted.

Management

Intubation and mechanical ventilation may be needed when patient fatigues and respiratory acidosis supervenes. Medical management should be continued. Tidal volume may have to be limited to 4–6 mL/kg with high inspiratory flow rates of 70–100 L/min to reduce the inspiratory time. Keep inspiratory plateau pressures below 30 cm H_2O with reduced I:E ratio of 1:3 or even lower to reduce air trapping. Positive end-expiratory pressure (PEEP) should be reduced if required to prevent hyperinflation. This all may lead to hypercapnia and acidosis initially. Again daily chest X-rays may be required.

Chronic Obstructive Pulmonary Disease

Diagnosis

Chronic obstructive pulmonary disease (COPD) can be classified into chronic bronchitis or emphysema depending upon the presentation. This presents with

cough, decreased exercise capacity, increased shortness of breath and sputum production, and fatigue. There is mild to moderate hypoxia and CO_2 retention leading to respiratory acidosis that is compensated by metabolic alkalosis. The mechanism is increased airway resistance that is chronic and only partially reversible differentiating it from asthma. There is also increased chances of viral and bacterial infections and altered lung mechanics. Differentiate from asthma, pneumonia, cardiac failure and musculoskeletal abnormalities.

Management

Severe exacerbation of COPD will lead to very low peak expiratory flow rate, acidosis with increased CO_2, right heart failure, pneumothorax, pneumonia, multiorgan failure and very poor response to therapy. Oxygen should be started at a low rate and medical therapy started as soon as possible with nebulised salbutamol and ipratropium bromide. Oral or intravenous steroids are used and then tapered over days. Antibiotics are recommended in suspected bacterial pneumonia with penicillin and macrolides to cover community acquired pneumonia. In some patients noninvasive ventilation is recommended and can reduce the hospital stay and avoid intubation in many cases. If severe respiratory failure, altered conciousness level and inability to tolerate noninvasive ventilation (NIV), mechanical ventilation after intubation may be needed. Many of these patients will need tracheostomies for weaning from mechanical ventilation.

Pulmonary Thromboembolism

Diagnosis

Pulmonary embolism results from formation of clot in the pulmonary artery and resulting in hampered blood flow through the pulmonary circulation. Patients experience dyspnea, tachycardia, tachypnea, chest pain, hypotension, syncope, cyanosis and refractory shock. The usual cause is deep vein thrombus migrating to the pulmonary bed. Hypoxia is present with increased A-a gradient, reduced $paCO_2$ due to increased ventilation. Sinus tachycardia is common, but right heart strain and typical 'S1Q3T3' sign may be present in rare cases. D-dimer, and fibrin degradation products may be elevated. Chest X-ray may be normal, but focal oligemia, small effusion and diaphragmatic hump may be present in some patients. Diagnosis is confirmed by CT pulmonary angiogram and Doppler of the leg veins may show deep vein thrombosis (DVT). Ventilation perfusion scans may be required if high suspicion and negative imaging. Risk factors include obesity, immobilization, previous DVT, recent surgery, malignancy, congestive heart failure and prothrombotic states. Differentiate from pneumonia, asthma, congestive heart failure and fat embolism.

Well's score can be used in defining the suspicion for pulmonary embolism (PE).
1. Clinical suspicion of DVT—3 points
2. Alternate diagnosis less likely—3 points
3. Tachycardia >100—1.5 points
4. Immobilization >3 days/surgery in last month—1.5 points
5. History of DVT or PE—1.5 points
6. Hemoptysis—1 points
7. Malignancy or palliative—1 points.

If the score is >4—Suspect PE and get imaging done

If the score is <4—PE less likely.

Management

Prevention is important and low molecular weight heparins should be used in any patient who is high-risk. Anticoagulation is recommended if DVT or PE is suspected and there is no hemodynamic compromise. Thrombolytic therapy is indicated if hemodynamic compromise is present with hypotension, right heart failure or cardiac arrest.

Air Embolism

Diagnosis

Signs and symptoms of air embolism are similar to a pulmonary thromboembolism; but the presentation is usually sudden with severe hypoxia, collapse, hypotension and increased right sided pressures occasionally leading to symptoms of stroke. This is most often iatrogenic with central venous lines the main culprit. This can occur during insertion or removal of central line or due to disconnection or accidental injection of air. Occasionally also seen in trauma with open veins, surgery, diving, hemodialysis, thoracotomy, bypass surgeries and surgeries where head up or sitting up position is used (neurosurgery, shoulder surgeries, ENT surgeries). Paradoxical emboli occurs due to presence of patent foramen ovale and increased right sided pressures leading to right to left shunting of air. The air bubbles can be visualized on echocardiography or occasionally on chest X-ray or CT scans. Differentiate from tamponade, pulmonary thromboembolism, myocardial infarction or anaphylaxis.

Management

If possible place the patient on the left side and head down to prevent air progressing further into the pulmonary circulation. If resulting from central venous access, the air can be aspirated. Supportive care with oxygen, fluid and cardiopulmonary resuscitation should be started. If air embolism suspected and no central venous access present, new line can be placed to remove air. Hyperbaric oxygen can be used to aid dissolution of air in blood. Caution on placement and removal of central line- always do it in head down position and keep all the ports well secured all the times.

Obstructive Sleep Apnea

Diagnosis

Obstructive sleep apnea presents as daytime sleepiness with obstruction in upper airway during sleep. The episodes of apnea last up to 90 seconds and terminate with wakening up due to hypoxia and sleep disturbance. Accessory muscles may be used during these episodes with intercostal retraction. Hypercapnia, hypoxia, and hemodynamic disturbances may be present and over time may lead to pulmonary and systemic hypertension. They may be associated with bradycardias and ectopic beats. This is more common in obese male patients with snoring, craniofacial abnormalities, airway edema and other obstructive lesions in the mouth. Differentiate from hypoventilation syndromes, and simple snoring.

Management

These cases should be evaluated in hospital with measurements of blood pressures and desaturations during sleep (polysomnography and sleep studies). Many patients will benefit from nasal continuous positive airway pressure (CPAP) in the night time. Oxygen therapy should be used with caution as they may increase the apneic episodes. Head end can be elevated or lateral position used during sleep. Intubation or tracheostomies can be used in patients known to have sleep apnea and prolonged admission in intensive care unit (ICU). Sedatives, hypnotics and opioids should be used with caution in such patients.

Obesity Hypoventilation Syndrome

Diagnosis

A central disorder leading to hypoventilation leading to presence of somnolence, lethargy and stupor due to respiratory acidosis and signs of right heart failure. Obstructive disease may be present along with this. Depression of respiratory stimulation to high $paCO_2$ is and low paO_2 is present along with increased work of breathing and abnormal lung and heart capacity. This is usually present in morbidly obese patients and leads to right heart failure and cor pulmonale. This can be associated with obstructive sleep apnea. Differentiate from drugs, obstructive sleep apnea (OSA), chronic obstructive pulmonary disease (COPD), hypothyroidism and cardiac failure.

Management

Many patients will need intubation and ventilation for this to improve oxygenation and reduction in CO_2. Over time the hypercapnic sensitivity may return. Noninvasive ventilation may be tried first before intubation and mechanical ventilation. Diuretics may be needed to reduce volume load along with other cardiac medications. Medroxyprogesterone acetate may be beneficial on the long-term therapy. Again avoid hypnotics and sedative agents and other opioids as they can suppress the respiratory drive further.

Aspiration Pneumonia

Diagnosis

Aspiration can result in chemical inflammation if gastric juices are aspirated and is called aspiration pneumonitis or infection with bacteria when its called aspiration pneumonia. Chemical irritation can lead to cough, wheeze, hypoxia and radiograph changes after 2–6 hours after the event. Bacterial infection will also lead to the above along with fever and signs of infection. Both can lead to acute respiratory distress syndrome and hypoxia. This is more common in patients having anesthetic, impaired conciousness, alcohol intake, critically ill patients, patients with nasogastric tubes and supine or head down positions. Differentiate from other causes of acute respiratory distress syndrome (ARDS), pulmonary edema, community or hospital-acquired pneumonia.

Management

Treat as respiratory failure and keep airway clear. In patients at high risk of aspiration during anesthesia, rapid sequence induction may reduce the incidence of aspiration. Aspiration pneumonitis do not need antibiotics unless they show signs of infection. Similarly steroids should be avoided. For suspected or confirmed aspiration pneumonia, antibiotics should be used. Antibiotics used for community acquired pneumonia are used if patients in hospital less than 3 days, while cover for gram-negative bacteria like *Pseudomonas* should be started if this is more than 3 days.

Ventilator-associated Pneumonia

Diagnosis

The diagnosis is made for patients on mechanical ventilation with fever, new lung infiltrates, raised white cell count and purulent secretions. This occurs in up to 25% of the mechanically ventilated patients and increases the mortality and duration of ventilation. The endotrachial or tracheostomy tube cuff are not full proof and microaspiration occurs around the cuff leading to oropharyngeal

bacteria causing pneumonia. Gram-negative bacilli, *Staphylococcus* and various other oral bacteria cause resistant pneumonia. Culture of sputum and blood should be sent when the diagnosis is suspected if possible with protected brushes, bronchoalveolar lavage or bronchoscopic samples. Differentiate from community acquired pneumonia, acute respiratory distress syndrome (ARDS) from other causes, pulmonary edema and pulmonary embolism.

Management

Aspirating the secretions and bronchoscopies if mucus plugging present and for sampling. Physiotherapy to drain secretions. Antibiotics should be directed towards the common organisms including gram-negative bacteria and possible cover for *Staphylococcus aureus*. The broad spectrum antibiotics can then be narrowed depending on the culture growth. The incidence can be reduced by following the ventilator care bundle which includes head up position, daily sedation hold, oral decontamination and toileting, supraglottic suction port in the endotracheal tubes and enteral feeds.

Hypoxia

Diagnosis

Hypoxia is defined as arterial PO_2 <60 mm Hg or saturations below 92% on room air, and also when the PaO_2 is less than expected with supplemental oxygen. This may present with tachypnea, tachycardia, sweating, anxiety, and cardiovascular compromise. Further deterioration may lead to confusion, drowsiness and coma. Type 1 respiratory failure is present when there is no retention of CO_2, but if retention is present it is called type 2 respiratory failure. Respiratory acidosis may be present leading to impaired consciousness. Causes include pneumonia, chronic obstructive pulmonary disease (COPD), asthma, embolism, acute respiratory distress syndrome (ARDS), lung fibrosis, effusions, edema, atelectasis, etc. Differentiate from low cardiac output states, shock, anemia, carboxyhemoglobinemia, high altitude, and methemoglobinemia.

Management

Control airway and breathing. Arterial blood gases are done to confirm the acid–base balance and compensation. Supplemental oxygen is started as soon as possible. Correct hypoxia to a minimum of 92% saturations or paO_2 >60 mm Hg. In chronic lung disease, care must be taken not to over correct the hypoxia as the respiratory drive may be dependent on hypoxia rather than the CO_2 levels in blood. These patients respond generally to lower FiO_2 as V/Q mismatch is present; while in ARDS, pneumonia and atelectasis, higher FiO2 is required due to the shunting. These patients may require intubation and ventilation in severe cases.

Hypercapnia

Diagnosis

Hypercapnia is said to be present when the $PaCO_2$ >45 mm Hg and respiratory acidosis is present. Patients may have headache, confusion, lethargy and coma. Hypoxia is simultaneously present will be defined as type 2 respiratory failure. Severe pulmonary disease may lead to hypercapnia, but this may be present with ventilatory insufficiency due to neuromuscular disorders and poisoning/overdose. Differentials include pulmonary disease like chronic obstructive pulmonary disease (COPD), interstitial lung disease, edema; neuromuscular disorder like Guillain-Barré syndrome (GBS), stroke, sedative overdose, head injury, myasthenia gravis, electrolyte problems, diaphragmatic injury and chest wall diseases.

Management

Establish airway and control breathing. Supplemental oxygen is usually needed in most cases. Arterial blood gas (ABG) should be done to assess the problem and compensation. Ventilation is usually required either noninvasive or invasive ventilation depending on the paitent or the cause. Treat the underlying cause once established.

Hemoptysis

Diagnosis

Bleeding into the pulmonary tree with expectoration of blood with coughing is a serious medical emergency. Common causes are infections including tuberculosis, aspergillosis, trauma, cardiovascular disorders like mitral stenosis and pulmonary edema and lung cancer. More than 600 mL of blood over 16 hours has a very high mortality if untreated. The bleeding is more if coagulopathy, infection, or renal failure is present. Arterial source is found in up to 90% patients. Differentiate from upper airway bleeding or upper gastrointestinal (GI) bleeding.

Management

Maintaining airway patency is paramount. Endotracheal intubation may be required if the bleeding is severe and causing cardiorespiratory compromise. If the source of bleeding is found and isolated in any particular lung, double lumen tube may be tried to restrict soiling and tamponading the source of bleeding. CT scan or bronchoscopy may localize the site of bleeding and occasionally may be controlled locally. Angiography may be tried and embolization attempted. Surgical advise should be sought early and may be needed in large number of patients. Underlying coagulation abnormalities should be treated along with infections.

Acute Respiratory Distress Syndrome

Diagnosis

Acute respiratory distress syndrome (ARDS) is defined as severe hypoxia that is refractory to supplemental oxygen with a PaO_2/FiO_2 ratio of less than 300. This should also be supported by diffuse infiltrates on chest X-ray with no evidence of congestive cardiac failure. Most of these patients will have sepsis, pneumonia, aspiration, trauma or pancreatitis, transfusion reaction, embolism, etc. The mortality remains high and increases if sepsis present on top of old age, multiple organ dysfunction, infection and renal failure. Differentiate from cardiogenic pulmonary edema, pneumonia or atelectasis.

Management

Treatment of the underlying cause should be started promptly. Patients will need high oxygen concentrations and most patients will need intubation and mechanical ventilation. High positive end expiratory pressures have to be used and low tidal volumes are useful in reducing mortality and morbidity while accepting high $paCO_2$. Fluids should be restricted as possible, but many patients will have long-term morbidity and mortality. ARDS net protocol can be followed once diagnosis is made to set the ventilator and determine the level of PEEP required.

Ventilation in ARDS

Concepts

The lung injury is diffuse and nonhomogeneous. Here the oxygenation goal should be to reach a paO_2 of 55 mm Hg by increasing the FiO_2 and positive end-expiratory pressure (PEEP) as needed. As a high FiO_2 on the long-term can lead to pulmonary toxicity, this should ideally be kept below 40–60% if possible. PEEP increases the endexpiratory volume and prevents lung collapse and atelectasis. Low volume ventilation strategy has been proven to be beneficial (Vt <6 mL/kg). This improves survival, prevents lung damage by barotraumas, but may lead to hypercapnia and acidosis.

Management

Tidal volume should be kept below 6 mL/kg while keeping the plateau pressure below 30 cm H_2O, if necessary with lower tidal volumes. Aim for normal pH though slight respiratory acidosis is acceptable. PEEP should be increased if the oxygen requirements are high to achieve PaO_2 >55 mm Hg. This can be increased till cardiovascular compromise is seen. Daily chest X-rays may be needed to rule out barotraumas and possible pneumothorax. The I:E ratios may have to be changes to 1:1 or rarely inversed to 2:1 to achieve sufficient oxygenation. Other modes of ventilation have been used like high frequency ventilation and prone positioning. These can improve the oxygenation in the short-term but may fail to offer any survival benefit. ECMO may be used for severe ARDS in selected cases.

Suggested Reading

1. Ferrer M, Bernadich O, Nava S, Torres A. Noninvasive ventilation after intubation and mechanical ventilation. Eur Respir J. 2002;19:959-65.
2. Heffner J, Brown L, Barbieri C. "Diagnostic value of tests that discriminate between exudative and transudative pleural effusions. Primary Study Investigators". Chest 1997;111(4):970-80.
3. http://www.ardsnet.org
4. Light RW. Pleural diseases (5th ed). Lippincott Williams & Wilkins. 2007;p. 310.
5. Mulgrew AT, Fox N, Ayas NT, Ryan CF. "Diagnosis and initial management of obstructive sleep apnea without polysomnography: a randomized validation study". Annals of Internal Medicine. 2007;146(3):157-66.
6. Raskin JM, Benjamine E, Iberti TJ. Venous air embolism: Case report and review. Mt Sinai J Med. 1985;52:367.
7. Shah R, Saltoun CA. "Chapter 14: Acute severe asthma (status asthmaticus)". Allergy and asthma proceedings: The Official Journal of Regional and State Allergy Societies. 2012;33 Suppl 1:S47-50.
8. Yap KS, Kalff V, Turlakow A, Kelly MJ. "A prospective reassessment of the utility of the Wells score in identifying pulmonary embolism". Med J Aust. 2007;187(6): 333-6.

Index

Page numbers followed by *f* refer to figure and *t* refer to table

A

Acetylcholine receptor 60
Acid-base
  balance 90
  disorders 90
Acidemia, severe symptomatic 91
Acid-fast bacilli 167
Acidosis 81, 103, 181
  chronic 54, 91
  lactic 90
  metabolic 47, 90
  respiratory 92, 93
Activated partial thromboplastin time 158, 172, 175
Acute respiratory distress syndrome 49, 63, 114, 132, 158, 164, 168, 187, 194, 195, 197
Addison's disease 80, 85
Adenoma, adrenal 107
Adrenal
  failure 105
  insufficiency 81, 85, 105
  steroids 107
Adrenocorticotropic hormone 106, 107
Agitation 15
Air embolism 1, 192
  signs of 192
  symptoms of 192
Airway 186
  obstruction 92
Akinetic mutism 76
Alanine transaminase 114, 124, 125, 131
Alcohol 18, 42
Alkaline phosphatase 124
Alkalosis 83, 85
  metabolic 91
  respiratory 93, 94
All-trans retinoic acid 110
Alopecia 155
American Diabetes Association 104
Amiodarone 34, 53
Amitriptyline overdose 54
Amniotic fluid embolism 114, 150
Amphetamines 51

Anaphylactoid reactions 101
Anemia 124, 155, 157, 181
  dilutional 181
  severe 29
Aneurysm 44
Angina 30, 37
  unstable 29, 30
Angiography 122
Antacids 26, 87
Anterior wall myocardial infarction 31*f*
Antibodies
  antinuclear 53, 156
  development of 60
Anticholinergics 74
Anticholinesterase inhibitors 61
Anticoagulation 12
Anticonvulsants 74
Antidepressants 74
Anti-neutrophil cytoplasmic antibodies 53, 153
Antiphospholipid syndrome 158
Anxiety 15, 94
  causes of 15
Aorta, coarctation of 44
Aortic
  dissection 41, 43, 44, 100
  hematomas 43*f*
  valve 39
Apthous oral ulcers 156
Arrythmias 3
Arterial blood gas 94, 195, 196
Artery rupture, pulmonary 11
Arthralgia 155, 156
Arthritis 155, 156
Ascites 126
Aspartate aminotransferase 51, 114, 124, 125, 131
Aspiration 194
  pneumonitis 22, 194
Asthma 99, 115, 189, 195
  acute severe 41, 189, 190
Ataxia 59
Atonic seizures 77
Atrial fibrillation 33-36, 44
  treatment of 35

Attacks, acute 116
Autoimmune disorders 157

B

Barbiturate 137
Bartter's syndrome 83, 92
Basal metabolic rate 183
Battle sign 65
Beck's triad 40
Becker disease 62
Becker dystrophy 61
Benzodiazepine 136, 137
    use of 18
Bicarbonate 104
    loss of 90
    retention 92
Bilevel positive airway pressure 189
Bleeding 14, 98, 176
    diasthesis 3
Blood
    loss 1, 99
    pressure 66
    stream infections 164
    sugar control 23
    transfusion 81
    urea nitrogen 46, 50, 125
Bloodstream infections 22
Botulism 59, 60, 62, 63, 169
Bowel obstruction 119
Bradycardia 32
Brain
    death 179
    injury 80, 100
        traumatic 67
Bristol stool chart 128*f*
Burns 25, 50, 81, 98, 150, 171, 179
Butterfly rash 155

C

Cachexia 63
Calcinosis 156
Calcium 111
    channel blocker overdose 133
    deficiency 84
    supplements 84
Campylobacter jejuni 58
    infection 59
Cancer 150
Candida albicans 171
Capnogram, normal 5*f*, 6*f*
Capnography 5
Capnometry 5
Carbon
    dioxide monitoring 5
    monoxide poisoning 138
Cardiac disease 183
    hypertensive 42

Cardiac failure 12, 47, 193
    congestive 42, 80, 168
Cardiac tamponade 40, 41*f*, 100
Cardiomyopathy 42, 98
    hypertrophic 39
    restrictive 41
Cardiovascular system 29
Catheter
    knotting of 11
    placement of 10
Central hyperventilation syndrome 93
Central nervous system 76, 132, 133, 144, 167
Central venous
    oxygen saturations 2
    pressure 2
Cerebral perfusion pressure 7, 67
Cerebrospinal fluid 58, 153
Charcot's triad of fever 129
Chest wall diseases 196
Chicken pox 147
    rash 147*f*
Chlamydia pneumoniae 163
Chloride resistant 92
Cholangitis
    acute 128
    ascending 128
Cholecystitis 114
Cholinergic crisis 61
Chronic obstructive pulmonary disease 64, 93, 94, 189, 190, 193, 195, 196
Churg-Strauss disease 53
Cirrhosis 80
Clonic seizures 77
Clonidine 21
Clostridium botulinum bacteria 169
Clostridium difficile 127, 163, 165, 166
    infections 165
Clostridium infection 170
Clostridium tetani bacteria 168
Cocaine 51
Colitis, ischemic 166
Coma 65, 75, 92
Complete blood count 66
Confusion 15, 181
Conn's syndrome 79, 92
Continuous positive airway pressure 187, 188, 193
Coronary artery disease 42
Corticosteroids 61
Corticotropin releasing hormone 106
Cough 111
Coxsackievirus 125
C-reactive protein 157
Creatine kinase 50, 141
Crest syndrome 156
Cullen's signs 124
Cushing's disease 107
Cushing's syndrome 91, 92, 106, 107
Cushing's triad 68

Cyanosis 112
Cystic fibrosis 91
Cytomegalovirus 58, 125, 182
   infections 160

D

Deep vein thrombosis 59, 73, 183, 191
Dehydration 74
Delirium 19
Dementia 74
Depression 18
Dexmedetomidine 21
Diabetes 29, 42, 85, 86, 183
   insipidus 79
   mellitus 90
Diaphoresis 15
Diaphragmatic injury 196
Diarrhea 22, 47, 80, 82, 90, 98, 127, 165
   noninfectious 166
   severe 79
Diphtheria 59
Diplopia 60
Discoid rash 156
Disseminated intravascular coagulation 76, 110, 114, 143, 147, 150, 158, 170, 172, 173, 175, 177, 178
Distress, causes of 15
Diuretics 80, 83, 112
   therapy 85
Dopamine agonists 74
Drug
   eruptions 170
   reactions 148, 152
   toxicity 47
Duchenne and Becker muscular dystrophy 61
Duke's criteria, classical 162
Duodenal ulcers 123
Duroziez sign 40
Dyslipidemia 29
Dysmotility 156
Dyspnea 15, 112

E

Eclampsia 113
   disorders, treatment of 85
Edema 112
   pulmonary 94, 116, 189
Edrophonium test 60
Ehler-Danlos syndrome 44
Electrical injuries 144
Electrolyte disorders 79
Embolism 1
   pulmonary 29, 44, 168, 183, 192
Emphysema, subcutaneous 14
Empyema 12
Encephalitis 167

Encephalopathy
   hepatic 67
   uremic 47, 54
Endocarditis 39
   infective 161
End-tidal carbon dioxide measurement 5
Entamoeba histolytica 165
Epilepsy 137
Epstein-Barr virus 182
Erythema multiforme 151
Erythrocyte sedimentation rate 157
Euvolemia 79
Extracorporeal membrane oxygenators 98

F

Fanconi's syndrome 86, 87
Fatigue 60, 155
Fatty liver, acute 114
Fever 94, 155
Fibrillatory waves 34
Fibrosis, pulmonary 93, 94
Fistula, bronchopleural 12
Flow directed pulmonary artery catheter 9
Fluid
   collection of 186
   depletion 47
   disorders 79
   overload 42, 47, 181
   replacement 103
   resuscitation 125
   therapy 47, 99
Fournier's gangrene 170
Fresh frozen plasma 177
Frostbite 142

G

Gabapentine 21
Gas gangrene 170
Gastric ulcer, prevention of 24
Gastritis 122
Gastroesophageal reflux 29
Gastrointestinal bleeding 166, 175, 196
Gitelman's syndrome 83, 92
Glasgow coma scale 65, 75
Glass test 153
Glomerulonephritis 47, 162
Glucocorticoids 54, 62, 112
Glucose control, methods of 24
Goiter 107
Goodpasture's syndrome 53, 157
Gordon's syndrome 81
Gower's sign 61
Graft versus host disease 152
Granulomas 157
Grave's disease 107, 108
Grey Turner signs 124
Guidewire stimulating heart 3

Guillain-Barré syndrome 58, 60, 62, 63, 92, 169, 196

H

Haemophilus influenzae 160, 163
Hashimoto's thyroiditis 108
Head injury 64, 196
Headache 15, 68, 111
Heart
   block 32
      rheumatic 39
      valvular 42
   failure 37, 42
      congestive 191
   rate 96
   sounds
      abnormal 38*f*
      normal 38*f*
   structures of 11*f*
Heatstroke 98, 141
Helicobacter pylori 24
HELLP syndrome 113, 114, 173
Hematoma 1, 3
Hematuria 155
Hemodialysis 2, 55, 86
Hemolysis 81, 85
Hemolytic uremic syndrome 173

Hemoptysis 157, 192, 196
Hemorrhage
   intracerebral 70*f*
   subarachnoid 67, 69, 71, 72
Hemothorax 3, 12
Hepatic failure 12, 25, 125
Hepatitis 125
Hepatorenal syndrome 52, 53
Hereditary defects 83
Heyde's syndrome 40
High thoracic spinal injury 100
Human immunodeficiency virus 167, 168
Hydralazine 54
Hydration 49
Hydrocephalus 67
Hyperaldosteronism 92
Hyperbilirubinemia 124
Hypercalcemia 83, 83*f*
Hypercapnia 91, 196
Hypercholesterolemia 44
Hyperglycemia 103
Hyperkalemia 47, 54, 81, 81*f*, 111, 181
Hypermagnesemia 85
Hypernatremia 79, 80
Hyperparathyroidism 85
   primary 84
   secondary 84
   tertiary 84
Hyperphosphatemia 85, 86, 111
   symptoms of 86

Hyperplasia 107
Hyperpnea 15
Hyperpyrexia, malignant 51
Hypersplenism 173
Hypertension 15, 29, 44, 91, 181, 183
   acute pulmonary 100
   intracranial 67
   pulmonary 155
Hyperthyroidism 84, 107
Hypertonia 77
Hypertonic saline 79
Hyperuricemia 111
Hyperventilation 85
   iatrogenic 94
Hypervolemia 54, 79, 88
Hypocalcemia 83*f*, 84, 181
Hypoglycemia 105, 137
   symptoms of 105
Hypokalemia 51, 82, 82*f*, 91, 92
Hypomagnesemia 83, 85, 86
Hyponatremia 80, 91
   correction of 80
   euvolemic 80
   hypervolemic 80
   hypovolemic 80
Hypoparathyroidism 84
Hypophosphatemia 51, 87
Hypotension 47, 91, 166, 181
Hypothalamic disorder 106
Hypothermia 108, 141, 142
Hypothyroidism 18, 80, 85, 108, 193
Hypovolemia 79, 88, 98
Hypoxia 93, 191, 195

I

Infarction, pulmonary 11
Infection 1, 12, 11, 14, 41, 74, 150, 159
Inhalational injury, acute 144
Intensive care unit 21, 23, 24, 48, 54, 64, 74, 79, 152, 160, 162-164, 171, 182, 186, 189
Intracranial pressure 7, 66, 67, 68*f*, 76, 79
   monitoring 7
   waves 9*f*
Intrauterine device 115

J

Janeway lesions 162
Jaundice 129

K

Kaposi's sarcoma 182
Kawasaki's disease 170
Ketamine 21, 137
Ketoacidosis 90
   diabetic 103, 104, 132
Ketoconazole 107

Ketonemia 104
Ketonuria 104
Kidney injury 46, 48, 49
Koplik's spots 146

L

Lactate dehydrogenase 51
Lambert-Eaton myasthenic syndrome 59, 60
Large bowel obstruction 119, 119f, 120
Leucocytosis 157
Leukemia, acute 110
Leukopenia 155
Liddle syndromes 92
Light's criteria 187
Listeria monocytogenes 160
Lithium intoxication 85
Liver
    dysfunction, drug-induced 114
    enzymes 125
    transplantation 53
Lung
    injury, acute 178
    parenchymal injury 14

M

Malabsorption 86
Malaise 156, 181
Malar rash 155, 156
Malnutrition 74
Marfan's syndrome 39, 44
Mean arterial pressure 7, 67
Measles 146, 170
    rash 146f
    virus 146
Mechanical ventilation 25, 99
Memory loss 15
Meningitis 137
    bacterial 166
Meningococcal infection 153, 166
Meningococcal rash 154f
Meningoencephalitis 72
Methanol
    ingestion of 90
    poisoning 134
Mifepristone 107
Migraine 72
Military tuberculosis 168
Milk alkali syndrome 84, 85
Miller Fisher syndrome 59
Mitral regurgitation 39
Mitral valve 38
Mixed acid-base disturbances 94
Molecular weight heparin, low 27, 73
Monro-Kellie doctrine 7, 67
Motor axonal neuropathy, acute 59
Motor neuron disease 60, 62, 92

Multifocal atrial tachycardia 34, 36
Multisystem
    disease 155
    failure 53
Mumps 125
Muscle
    biopsy 61
    relaxants 92
    specific tyrosine kinase antibodies 60
Muscular dystrophies 61
Musculoskeletal pain 29
Myasthenia 61
    gravis 59, 60, 62, 92, 93, 196
Myasthenic crisis 61
Mycobacterium tuberculosis 167
Mycoplasma 58, 125
Myeloid leukemia, acute 110
Myeloma, multiple 84
Myocardial infarction 30, 31f, 42, 44, 98
Myoclonic jerks 77
Myoclonic seizures 77
Myopathy 63, 64
Myositis 51
Myxedema 108
Myxoma 162
    atrial 39, 162

N

Nasal endotracheal tubes 159
Nasogastric tube 22, 26, 159
Nausea 68, 155, 181
Necrosis 148
Necrotizing fasciitis 169
Neisseria meningitidis 153
Nephrotic syndrome 80, 155
Nerve conduction studies 58, 63
Nervous system 157
Neuroleptic malignant syndrome 51
Neuromuscular diseases 92
Neurosurgery 192
Nikolsky's sign 150
Noninvasive ventilation 188, 188f, 191
Nonsteroidal anti-inflammatory drugs 143, 150, 159, 174, 181
Nutrition 21

O

Obesity 29
    hypoventilation syndrome 93, 193
Obstructive sleep apnea 108, 193
Ophthalmoplegia 59
Opioid 21, 74, 92, 136, 137
Oral condidiasis 153f
Osler nodes 162
Oxygen supplementation 190
Oxygenation 66, 114, 186

P

Pain 1, 14, 20, 94
    abdominal 129, 155
    issues 15
    treatment of 20
Palpitations 15
Pancreatitis 84, 124
Papillary muscle rupture 39
Paralytic ileus 120, 120*f*
Parathyroid function, abnormal 84
Parenchymal disease 155
Partial thromboplastin time 175
Pemphigus vulgaris 151, 151*f*
Penicillamine 53
Peptic ulcer disease 25, 29, 123
Pericardial effusion 181
Pericarditis 29, 41, 44
    constrictive 41, 100
    uremic 47, 54
Peritoneal dialysis 55, 55*f*
Phosphate 111
    binders 87
Photoplethysmography 4
Photosensitivity 156
Pituitary adenoma 107
Plasma
    glucose 104
    transfusions 177
Plasmapheresis 2, 59, 158
Platelet dysfunction 181
    qualitative 174, 175
Pneumocystis jirovecii 160
    pneumonia 168
Pneumonia 132, 163, 195
    atypical 168
    community acquired 163, 195
    hospital-acquired 163
    ventilator associated 194
Pneumothorax 3, 12, 41, 185, 185*f*
Poisoning 54, 108, 130, 132, 142
    organophosphorus 93, 130
Poliomyelitis 59, 62
Polyangiitis, microscopic 53
Polydipsia, primary 80
Polymyositis 62
Polyneuropathy 63
Polysomnography 193
Positive end-expiratory pressure 187, 197
Post-parathyroidectomy surgery 85
Preeclampsia 113, 114
Pregnancy 26, 94, 113, 115
Pressure
    control ventilation 189
    monitoring 1, 2
    regulated volume control 189
    support ventilation 189
    time curve 187*f*

Procainamide 53
Promyelocytic leukemia, acute 110
Prostate enlargement 47
Protein deficiency 42
Proteinuria 155
Prothrombin time 172, 175, 176
Proton pump-inhibitor 25, 26
Psychosis 155, 156
Ptosis 60
Pulmonary artery catheter 2, 10*f*
    placement 9
Pulmonary function tests 116
Pulse 99
    oximetry 4, 5
    volume 99
Pupillary signs 65
Pyomyositis 62

Q

Quincke's pulse 40
Quinidine 53

R

Raccoon eyes 65
Raynaud's phenomenon 155
Red cell transfusion 176
Refeeding syndrome 22, 23, 86
Reflux 156
Regurgitation 156
Renal
    disorders 46
    dysfunction 156
    failure 12, 25, 48, 54, 85, 132, 157, 181
    function, abnormal 176
    injury, acute 54
    replacement 54
        therapy 2, 48, 54, 56*f*
    tubular acidosis 81, 86
Respiration rate 99
Respiratory failure 183
Reye's syndrome 125
Reynaud's disease 156
Reynold's pentad 129
Rhabdomyolysis 50, 63, 81, 85
Rheumatic disease 162
Richmond agitation and sedation scale 16, 16*t*
Roth spots 162
Rumack-Matthew nomogram 131*f*

S

Salicylate toxicity 94
Sarcoidosis 84
Scarlet fever 170
Scleroderma 152, 156
Sclerosis, systemic 156

Seizures 50, 155
    types of 77
Selective serotonin reuptake inhibitors 19
Sepsis 25, 47, 74, 84, 96, 137, 160, 161, 170
    neutropenic 161
    severe 96
Septal defect, atrial 39
Serositis 156
Serum-ascites albumin gradient 127
Sexually transmitted diseases 115
Shock 25, 96
    anaphylactic 101
    cardiogenic 97
    hypovolemic 98
    neurogenic 100
    obstructive 99
    septic 96, 161
    stages of 99, 99*t*
Shoulder surgeries 192
Sinus
    arrhythmia 34
    bradycardia 32*f*
    tachycardia 36
Skeletal muscles 60
Skin
    diseases 146
    pigmentation 5
    thickening 156
Small bowel obstruction 118, 118*f*
Snakebite 139
Sodium
    bicarbonate 82
        infusion 79
    fractional excretion of 50, 52
Spinal cord transection 59
Spirononlactone 81
Stable angina pectoris 29
Staphylococcus aureus 148, 162, 164, 195
Staphylococcus bacteriae 162
Status epilepticus 77
Stenosis
    aortic 39, 40
    mitral 38
Steroid deficiency 80
Steven-Johnson syndrome 148, 149, 152, 170
Stomach 123
Streptococci pneumoniae 163
Streptococci viridians 162
Streptococcus pneumoniae 166, 167
Streptococcus pyogenes 148
Streptococcus viridians 162
Stress 29
    ulcers 24
Stroke 67, 69, 72, 74, 92, 94, 176, 196
    hemorrhagic 69
    ischemic 69
    thromboembolic 69

Succinylcholine, use of 81
Sudden death 37
Superior vena cava syndrome 111
Sweating 79
Synchronized intermittent mandatory
    ventilation 189
Syncope 37
Syndrome of inappropriate antidiuretic
    hormone secretion 80
Syphilis 44
Systemic lupus erythematosus 53, 60, 152,
    155, 158

T

Tachycardia 15, 91, 192
    junctional 36
    supraventricular 35, 36, 36*f*
    ventricular 11, 36, 37, 37*f*
Tachypnea 96
Telangiectasias 156
Tension pneumothorax 99
Tetanus 51, 168
Thiazide diuretics 84
Thoracic deformities 93
Thrombocytopenia 150, 155, 157, 173
    heparin induced 173, 174
Thromboelastography 172
Thromboembolism, pulmonary 191
Thrombophilia 27
Thrombophlebitis 162
Thrombosis 1
Thrombotic thrombocytopenic purpura 150,
    173
Thymectomy 61
Thyroid disorders 42
Thyroiditis 107
Thyrotoxicosis 86, 107
Tonic-clonic seizures 77
Toxic epidermal necrolysis 149
    syndrome 148, 149, 151, 152
Toxic shock syndrome 148, 170
Toxins 42
Tracheostomy 62
Transfusion
    concepts of 177
    reactions 150, 178
Transjugular intrahepatic portosystemic
    shunt 53
Trauma 41, 44, 80, 98
Traumatic muscular damage 50
Tricuspid regurgitation 39
Tricyclic antidepressant 132-134
    poisoning 132
Tubular necrosis, acute 47, 49, 52
Tumor lysis syndrome 85, 111

U

Ulcer prophylaxis 25
Underwater seal systems, types of 13*f*
Universal pain assessment tool 20*f*
Upper airway obstruction 189
Upper gastrointestinal bleeding 121
Uremia 41
Uric acid 111
Urinary tract infection 162
Urine
    alkalinization of 111
    chloride 92
Urticaria 155

V

Valvular abnormalities 98, 162
Varicella 58
Vascular injury 11
Vasculitis 155, 157
Ventricular septal defect 39

Viral
    encephalitis 167
    exanthema 170
    infection 146, 152
Vital capacity, monitoring of 60
Vocal cord palsy 189
Volume control ventilation 189
Vomiting 47, 68, 80, 82, 98
von Willebrand's disease 175, 177
von Willebrand's factor 175

W

Warfarin toxicity 176
Water hammer pulse 40
Wegener's granulomatosis 53, 157
Well's score 192
Wenckebach's phenomenon 32
West Nile virus 167
Whipple's triad 105
White cell count 96, 124, 129, 160, 165, 166, 170
World Federation of Neurosurgeon's Grading 72*t*